Praise for *Coproduction: Towards equality in mental healthcare*

'Coproduction is on everyone's lips it seems, yet few really practise it, let alone do it well. This is particularly frustrating from a service user perspective, as the possibilities to totally transform mental healthcare are endless. This book is a welcome friend to reassure and inform your thinking and practice. Coproduction, put simply, is a way of being with people to work things out. If we do this in mental healthcare, we can not only change an awful structural power dynamic, we can actually get to the nub of people's issues. This book is joyous as it takes you through a variety of coproduction journeys, focusing on many rich experiences. There is plenty to explain what helps and hinders coproduction, and it also has an eye to a future of possibilities. This book gives me hope.'

Tina Coldham, mental health user consultant and survivor researcher

'Those of us working on the theory and practice of coproduction hanker after books that dig down into its implications in different fields, in a critical way. This book is supremely valuable in this regard. It is the first book-length treatment of coproduction in mental health – an area where it has distinct and powerful potential. As the editors rightly argue, that potential cannot be adequately gauged without taking on board the value basis of a kind of practice that prioritises inclusion and agency, and requires collaboration from the start, and 'all the way down'. Coproduction is about relationships, and what shines through the chapters in this book is a critical, engaged, resourceful and consistently imaginative sense of how those relationships go, in different settings and in connection with a range of differently situated individuals. What helps and hinders such relationships? What standards should apply to them? Who benefits, and how? How are they navigated, by practitioners, service users and carers? And how can we translate insights in these areas into future policy and practice? The book provides rich, unique and critically informed commentaries on all these questions, and more besides. It will provide a welcome and illuminating resource for anyone with an interest in what coproduction is and what it can offer.'

Dr Gideon Calder, Associate Professor, School of Social Sciences, Swansea University

'Coproduction is about bringing people together, forming meaningful relationships and addressing power imbalances. It is rarely easy and often challenging. This book brings together a diversity of authors to share their experiences and highlight the challenges and opportunities of coproduction in mental health services. In so doing, it provides an inspirational vision for a more inclusive future for mental health services. This needs to be read both by people who use services and those who provide them, to open up new possibilities for mental health care and support.'
Martin Webber, Professor of Social Work, University of York

'This book is fabulous, showcasing ways that coproduction works, with examples from all corners of mental health services, ranging from forensic to community, voluntary and social enterprise to mainstream NHS, research, learning disability and more. It is essential reading for those interested in what coproduction is and how it might be done, providing a vital addition to the scholarship on the subject. As these chapters demonstrate, where services are designed from the bottom up in non-hierarchical systems, the process becomes joyous, enriching and well worth the effort. Coproduction is not a zero-sum game, it is synergistic, and everyone involved gets more out than they put in.'
Dr Melvin Bradley, CEO, Mental Health Independent Support Team, Bolton

Coproduction:
Towards equality in mental healthcare

Edited by
Julian Raffay, Don Bryant, Pamela Fisher,
Mick McKeown, Catherine Mills and Tim Thornton

First published 2022

PCCS Books Ltd
Wyastone Business Park
Wyastone Leys
Monmouth
NP25 3SR
United Kingdom

contact@pccs-books.co.uk
www.pccs-books.co.uk

This collection ©Julian Raffay, Don Bryant, Pamela Fisher, Mick McKeown, Catherine Mills and Tim Thornton, 2022
The individual chapters © the contributors, 2022

All rights reserved.

No part of this publication may be reproduced, stored in a retrieval system, transmitted or utilised in any form by any means, electronic, mechanical, photocopying or recording or otherwise, without permission in writing from the publishers.

The authors have asserted their right to be identified as the authors of this work in accordance with the Copyright, Designs and Patents Act 1988.

Coproduction: Towards equality in mental healthcare

British Library Cataloguing in Publication data: a catalogue record for this book is available from the British Library.

ISBNs   paperback – 978 1 915220 03 5
         epub – 978 1 915220 04 2

Cover design by Hugh Cowling
Typeset in-house by PCCS Books using Minion Pro and Myriad Pro
Printed in the UK by Severn, Gloucester

CONTENTS

Introduction   *1*
Julian Raffay, Mick McKeown and Tim Thornton

SECTION 1
Navigating coproduction: Exploring the context of coproduction in services

Navigating coproduction: Introduction   *13*
Julian Raffay and Pamela Fisher

1   Towards the ideal ward round: A coproduced service improvement project   *18*
Gemma Stacey, Anne Felton, involvement volunteers and members of the Ideal Ward Round Steering Group

2   Mental health recovery through coproduction: African and Caribbean men's experiences in the United Kingdom   *31*
Kris Southby, Frank Keating and Stephen Joseph

3   Collaboration in secure care: A history of the past, the present and the future   *43*
Mark Chandley and AB

4   From depression to delight and nearly everything in between: A non-academic perspective   *58*
Elaine Harrison

Navigating coproduction: Conclusion   *66*
Julian Raffay and Pamela Fisher

SECTION 2
Barriers and facilitators to coproduction

Barriers and facilitators to coproduction: Introduction   *71*
Catherine Mills and Mick McKeown

5   Relational spaces for mental health and wellbeing   *76*
Rhiannon Corcoran, Maureen Thomas and Julia Zielke

6   Coproduction and care planning   *89*
Catherine Mills

7	Coproduction and addiction *Lucy Webb and Amanda Clayson*	102
8	Coproduction in forensic learning disability settings *Michaela Thomson, Mike Hargreaves and Shaun Peterson*	115
9	Breaking down the barriers to coproduction *Kate Pieroudis*	127

Barriers and facilitators to coproduction: Conclusion — 142
Mick McKeown and Catherine Mills

SECTION 3
Coproducing the future

Coproducing the future: Introduction — 147
Tim Thornton

10	A personal story and thoughts *Don Bryant*	152
11	Challenging co-option: From coproduction by organisations to co-creation of value by users *Andrew Passey*	163
12	The ethics of coproduction: Stumbling across the light *Julian Raffay and Walid Elkharam*	175
13	Coproducing democratic relationships *Mick McKeown, Albert Dzur and Pamela Fisher*	190

Coproducing the future: Conclusion — 202
Don Bryant

Conclusions — 206
David Pilgrim

Contributors — 215

Name index — 225

Subject index — 231

Acknowledgements

A huge thank you to Catherine Jackson and her colleagues at PCCS Books, who have worked alongside us throughout the production process. Catherine's supportive and unflappable approach and the expertise of PCCS Books have put a challenging task within reach.

Thank you to all who have given their time. Particular thanks to Amanda Rowlands for her invaluable contributions to the work of the editorial team. We are most grateful to those who have taken part in focus groups – without you, several chapters could not have been written. A special thank you to the contributors in secure services, who have had to write anonymously. We very much wanted to respect your right to be credited in your own names, and hope this may become possible in future publications.

Organising our meetings without a budget was a huge challenge. Thankfully, Mersey Care NHS Foundation Trust paid volunteers' expenses and enabled unwaged participants to attend.

We would like to thank the printer, distributors, librarians and course leaders who have made this book accessible. Finally, thank you for picking it up and reading it! We hope you find it as inspiring, challenging and stimulating as we have in compiling it.

About the editors

Julian Raffay was working as Specialist Chaplain (Research, Education and Development) until his post at Mersey Care was cut in March 2020. Since then, he has completed his professional doctorate on the relationship between mental health services and faith communities with particular emphasis on the ethics of coproduction. He returned briefly to church ministry as Interim Team Rector in an economically disadvantaged parish in Liverpool. He is now Director of Chaplaincy Studies at St Padarn's Institute, Cardiff.

Don Bryant was formerly a bank manager, set up a management training company with diverse clients across north-west England, joined Imagine, a Liverpool-based mental health charity, established an educational, training and employment centre for recovering drug users, and then became ill with severe depression in 2008. Since 2009 he has acted in numerous capacities as a service user and carer representative, winning the Chairman's Award in 2015. He also served as a trustee of the national Mental Health Network.

Pamela Fisher is an independent researcher. Until May 2019, she was a Reader in Social & Health Citizenship at Leeds Beckett University, having previously held academic posts at the universities of Sheffield, Huddersfield, Liverpool and Leeds. Her work offers critical sociological perspectives on resilience, wellbeing and mental health, particularly from the perspectives of marginalised and socially under-valued groups.

Mick McKeown is Professor of Democratic Mental Health, School of Nursing, University of Central Lancashire and a trade union activist with UNISON, playing a role in union strategising on professional nursing. He has published widely in the mental health field, including co-editing the recent textbook, *Essentials of Mental Health Nursing*.

Catherine Mills has worked as Service User and Carer Lead with Mersey Care NHS Foundation Trust since 2012, where she is responsible for the engagement and involvement of service users and carers across Merseyside. Originally she was involved with the trust as a service user. Her current role includes research, where she has been involved in several projects that have been coproduced with service users and carers.

Tim Thornton is Professor of Philosophy and Mental Health in the School of Nursing, University of Central Lancashire. As well as contemporary philosophy of thought and language, his research mainly concerns conceptual issues in mental healthcare, and he has published papers on clinical judgement, idiographic and narrative understanding, the interpretation of psychopathology and recovery, as well as numerous books. He was a co-editor of the *Oxford Handbook of Philosophy and Psychiatry* and is a senior editor of the journal *Philosophy, Psychiatry and Psychology*.

Introduction

Julian Raffay, Mick McKeown and Tim Thornton

If you read this book, please bring to it your unique personality, gifts and background. We have tried to write with you in mind, because you, like us, are an expert in your own experience. Our experience arises through engagement with the world and with others. And, as you read, our worlds meet – yours and ours.

We hope that, as you read the accounts we have assembled, you will do so less as a student and more as a friend, a kindred spirit. We need your friendship, for we have been honest to the point of fearing rejection, but please do not hesitate to be a critical friend. We have put ourselves on the line because we are committed to lighting up the dark recesses of mental health services through genuine friendship, respect and human warmth.

Indeed, friendship, respect and human warmth are probably more powerful than models, constructs and ideas. It is the former that have enriched our lives over the three years that we editors and authors have worked together, compiling the book you have before you.

As you read each chapter and the supporting material, imagine yourself – if you can do so without undue distress – in the situations described. Imagine yourself a service user, carer or member of staff (or each in turn). By all means, consider and weigh up the ideas you read. But please also take time with your feelings, your reactions and consider our invitation to embrace coproduction in your life and relationships.

We seek your forgiveness where our terminology offends or where we may have accidentally used discriminatory language. This was never our intention, although we have sometimes had to settle on a phrase for ease of communication or simplicity, or to allow an author to express things in their own words. We have used the words 'service user' and 'patient' as we find both are chosen by different people in receipt of mental health services. However, we recognise that neither phrase is in keeping with the book's democratising intent and that both ignore Kara's (2013, p.131) observation that we have more 'mutable identities'.

Responding to human distress

We begin this introduction by exploring coproduction in mental health services. We chose the heading 'responding to human distress' as a reminder that much of what is labelled 'mental health' may have its roots in disadvantage, neglect and abuse. As you read, do weigh up the assumptions the authors make; we have, in the spirit of coproduction, exercised the lightest possible editorial control.

The democratic ideal of coproduction has been suggested to redeem many existing problems in mental health services, not least difficulties that arise because of distinct power imbalances in favour of practitioners over service users. Mental health services, perhaps more than other healthcare arenas, are notable for their controversies. Many people who use these services have unproblematic, satisfactory or welcome experiences of sanctuary or healing. Many others, however, find their experiences of services so challenging that they refer to themselves as survivors (of the service, not the illness). Criticisms of services focus on aspects of compulsion and coercion and the powerfully controlling influence of bio-psychiatric orthodoxy. Coproduction joins a long list of organisational innovations that have, over the years, been offered to reform or even transform psychiatry and services. The jury is out on whether coproduction can fulfil this redemptive role.

It is our view that mental distress is such an important social issue that service provision to relieve it should be available. Yet the form this takes need not be limited by the psychiatric services we know now. Indeed, we would much rather see a range of services more in tune with the diverse demands that might be made of them by people with equally diverse needs. We hope that models of coproduction need not be constrained by a weight of heavy expectation, that they can revolutionise psychiatry as we know it. There is potential for transformation, and we feel this should be grasped, nurtured and sustained, to see how much progress can be made within current systems. To decry possible failure to achieve meaningful change without attempting it first is to be, as Peter Sedgwick (1982) said, the most adamant of conservatives. Not to act is simply to be complicit in leaving things as they are or, in Chandley and AB's words (see Chapter 5), indolence.

We feel that, even if entrenched psychiatric power proves insurmountable, there are many ways in which multiple efforts to enact ideals of coproduction might improve services. We may be able, on a smaller scale, to show new ways of providing mental healthcare that serve as models for larger-scale alternatives. The increasing democratisation of relationships within services might also be an end in itself. It might both point to an ideal of more equal relationships within less oppressive circumstances and concurrently improve the experiences of service users and staff. Seemingly small gains ought not to be criticised, as they can hold open the possibility of aggregating together. They might prefigure shaping the services we would like to see or provide a glimpse of some utopian future configuration. Improved democratic therapeutic relations may also hold the promise of enabling the trust and recognition necessary to build the political alliances we may need if we are to truly campaign and build for alternatives.

Even if all of this proves a self-deluded route to dilution and colonisation, we may be able to establish alternative social forms of service and support outside of the mainstream (Barker, 2003).[1] Arguably, most people can agree that coproduction ideals should form the basis for such organisations.

What is coproduction?

The New Economics Foundation defines coproduction as 'a relationship where professionals and citizens share power to design, plan and deliver support together, recognising that both partners have vital contributions to make to improve quality of life for people and communities' (Slay & Stephens, 2013, p.3). Affirming 'vital' contributions on both sides suggests we can enjoy coproduction without condemning the professionals. Coproduction merely asks that service users and carers be taken seriously as well.

However, there are weaknesses in Slay and Stephens' model. We might liken it to a sound system's volume control – the louder, the better. This image is useful, as Arnstein's ladder of participation underpins their approach. It has three progressive coproduction rungs (or volume levels): 'doing to', 'doing for', and 'doing with' (Arnstein, 1969; Slay & Stephens, 2013, p.3). Sadly, they gloss over Arnstein's (1969, pp.217, 224) nuanced perspective. An example illustrates the problem well: prisoners sewing mailbags fits Slay and Stephen's highest level, 'doing with', but involves compulsion.

A better image of coproduction might be a graphic equaliser (separately controlling the volumes of different frequencies) or multiple ladders (Tritter & McCallum, 2006, p.163). We prefer Mudhoni's richer perspective, which declares 'that participation is a complex and interactive process [...] that is

---

1. In this context, colonisation refers to the process where people in power adopt and dilute radical ideas to their own advantage.

essentially political in nature and takes place in a broader political context' (Mudhoni, 2014, p.31). Engaging this broader context calls for more strategic thinking than merely increasing the volume. We suggest it is better to coproduce our vision, work out vital contributions together, and then identify what we can achieve collectively (Tritter & McCallum, 2006, p.165).

We are increasingly convinced we need not just to coproduce but also to co-evaluate services. Staniszewska and colleagues remark (2012):

> The outcomes of involvement seemed to be predominantly defined by the organisations involved rather than service users, so we know relatively little about the outcomes that service users wanted to achieve. Such difficulties challenge the notion of true partnership as certain groups dominate the ways in which methods, context or process are decided. (p.138)

Responding to the hopes of service users calls for something more complicated than what our graphic equaliser represents. Thankfully, Tritter and McCallum's 'mosaic' model (2006) suggests 'that for user involvement to improve health services, it must acknowledge the value of the process and the diversity of knowledge and experience of both health professionals and lay people' (p.156). Their perspective discourages us from applying predetermined formulae, or even templates. Instead, coproduction invites us to relate to other people, which may be challenging but offers many advantages.

Why coproduction?

Mental health services do not exist in a vacuum. We need to understand the interest in coproduction against declining respect for professions and increasing rejection of medical paternalism (Schön, 1984, p.13; Department of Health, 2006, p.19; Baxter et al., 2010; Cooke, 2014, p.104). Austerity and growing bureaucratic complexity point to the need for a new approach, perhaps even more pressing as we contemplate new futures beyond current crises, of which the Covid-19 pandemic is perhaps the most significant. What Church and Reville (1989) described in Canada more than 30 years ago is strikingly familiar:

> As reliance on institutional responses becomes ever more expensive, and as health status bears less and less relationship to expenditure, governments and societies will face a difficult choice. Either they will cling to traditional approaches and contain costs by rationing services or they will develop new approaches and shift more of the responsibility for health onto the shoulders of those who would be healthy. (1989, p.24)

That the business world makes so much of consumer experience gives us reason to believe it may be significant in healthcare provision (Pine II, 1999, p.6). Coproduction may promise better services but, when we consider its background, we discover that greater user representation of itself does not guarantee better services. That demands genuine 'relationship' (Slay & Stephens, 2013, p.3). Where service users, carers and staff plan, deliver and evaluate together, there should be better protection from disastrous failure, such as occurred in Mid-Staffordshire (Francis, 2013, p.4).

Arguments against coproduction

Inertia is not organisations' only reason for avoiding coproduction. We can expect four main charges to be levelled: naïve optimism, difficulties measuring outcomes, mental capacity and expense. On the charge of naive optimism, we readily accept that coproduction calls for courage. However, the system that the Schizophrenia Commission described as 'broken and demoralised' (2012, p.3) needs transforming if it is not to continue harming service users, carers and staff alike. Inevitably, those fearing loss of influence may be the first to raise this specific charge. We should not be naive about subtle manipulation and social processes (Hui & Stickley, 2007, p.424).

A second charge concerns how we might measure coproduction. We reach into ever-deeper waters as we move from the simplicity of Slay and Stephens' (2013) model to Tritter and McCallum's mosaic (2006). However, many service users want a service that is less focused on the measurable (Forrest et al., 2000). What nurses term 'patients' needs' may be mere projections of their own anxieties and may have little to do with patients' actual priorities. Horgan offers an example when she suggests that reducing cutting may not be the top priority for people who self-harm (2012, pp.131–132).

The third charge has to do with mental capacity. Many service users, carers and clinicians see human distress as having social and environmental causes (Os et al., 2010, p.210). Hubble and colleagues (1999, p.431) found recovery as much in the service user's control as anyone else's. Coproduction does not merely empower the service user; it also restores responsibility. In doing so, it debunks technocratic solutions, not least the assumption that managers understand the outcomes of their actions (Storm & Edwards, 2013, p.322).

Finally, we acknowledge that significant upfront costs are likely in advancing an organisation towards coproduction. We completely agree that financial arguments should inform choices. At the same time, excessive focus on the balance sheet can prevent us from recognising wider issues. Oliver, Kothari and May's *The Dark Side of Coproduction* (2019) helpfully uncovers hidden costs that deserve consideration. However, they ignore the possibility that service users and carers might want a quite different kind of service. If coproduction were truly effective in meeting need, it could end the distressing (and wasteful) 'revolving door' phenomenon (where most inpatient bed occupancies are readmissions). We hope that our book goes some way to refute Oliver, Kothari and May's contention that 'there is so little empirical evidence about how coproduction changes research, policy or practice, or how it may compare to alternatives' (2019, p.7). The most contentious issue of all concerns who sets the criteria for service evaluation. The NHS Constitution (Department of Health and Social Care, 2015) asserts that 'the NHS belongs to the people' (2015, p.2). The empirical evidence for that assertion is decidedly patchy; the contrary evidence sometimes feels overwhelming.

What we have learned

We have undoubtedly learned most about coproduction through the action of coproducing together. Unsurprisingly, we have learnt to respect disagreement and have worked towards the sort of mutual understanding noted by Lencioni (2002). We have had to invest time in one another to get beyond the often-competitive, superficial relationships that characterise many dysfunctional NHS teams. Having done so, however, we have saved time overall. We genuinely look forward to meeting as we support one another in advancing our work. Our approach has made effective use of time, but, more than that, the resulting friendship, respect and human warmth have been deeply therapeutic on all sides.

A big challenge has been organising our meetings without a budget. We had difficulty finding an accessible, affordable venue. We also faced challenges with NHS trust policies on data protection in relation to communication between service users and those outside the organisation. Our biggest headaches involved online collaboration. NHS protocols and hardware meant we could only use email to begin with. Latterly, the pandemic accelerated the welcome adoption of a range of digital forms of communication to usefully supplement or substitute for face-to-face meetings.

Our contribution

We warmly commend our book to you as we believe we are the first to coproduce a book on coproduction in mental health. Our self-reflexive approach resembles that of ethnographers. We are concerned to be deeply personal and relational and analytic, as we see this leading to better services and collective wellbeing. Although many have advocated coproduction, its open-ended nature makes it hard to evaluate through randomised controlled trials. We therefore see ethics as supplying a stronger argument than health economics (see Chapter 12). In particular, we hold that 'non-coproducing' traditionally delivered services should be considered deficient. Moreover, we challenge those who think otherwise to argue the case for their position.

We affirm the invaluable contribution made by the survivor movement (Survivors History Group, 2012) and we welcome a mixed economy. Alongside the survivor movement, we look to a place where staff who are open about their lived experience (and those who are sympathetic) can work alongside service users and carers in the pursuit of better services and beyond. Our experience has shown us that collaborative approaches can reach places that more adversarial approaches cannot. Ultimately, we need to be practical and balance criticality.

Our editorial team

To briefly explain how we (the editors) came together to create this book, we trace our origins back to some research conducted by Walsh and colleagues (2013) in Sheffield. They found that staff dismissed matters service users considered vitally important, and so set up a group to advocate for their concerns. Sheffield's Spirituality Strategy Group inspired Julian's doctoral research into coproduction (Raffay, 2020). When he moved to Mersey Care, he met like-minded service users, carers and staff. Together, they felt moved to write this book and formed the Coproduction Editorial Team. We are now a group of nine people committed to service transformation.

Many of us appear male, pale and quite possibly stale, but most, and possibly all, of us have suffered human distress at various stages in our lives. Several of us have used or – if you prefer – survived mental health services. We have made genuine efforts to achieve diversity and have, we think, succeeded to a degree. Again, our apologies if we have not addressed your situation. No promises, but we are open to the possibility of a second volume, so do let us know if you have a contribution to make.

Like any group, we faced many challenges along the way and patience was certainly a necessary virtue! The hardest decisions were around editorial control. Too much exercise of power would have stood in the way of coproduction. Neglect of our responsibilities would have left the authors out on a limb without support. You will see that we have chosen a light touch, but we stand by the authors, many of whom have showed remarkable courage. We particularly stand by the novice authors and hope you will enjoy the freshness of their work.

This collection has been in part influenced by an Economic and Social Research Council (ESRC) seminar series (principal investigator, Pamela Fisher) in 2016 and 2017. The starting point of this series was that everyone – service users, carers, professionals and academics – has something to contribute, and that this requires everyone to engage in deep and reflective listening, accompanied by a readiness to learn from each other, rather than merely to defend deeply held assumptions.

The structure of the book

The book is in three sections. The first was originally named 'Successes in Coproduction' but we renamed it 'Navigating Coproduction' because we wanted to share honest experiences and avoid the hype so common in marketing ideas and products. By being honest, we hope the book will better help you light up dark places. In this first section, the authors offer a broad foundation for understanding coproduction. Readers already familiar with the topic may enjoy making connections between their context and the diverse settings we explore. Section 2 continues to narrate experiences but with an emphasis on barriers and facilitators. The contributors share accounts of the challenges they met and how they overcame them. Section 3 explores futures that may emerge through the practice of coproduction. Since coproduction is, by its very nature, open ended, we deliberately avoid being in any way prescriptive.

Critical issues to consider

In a book of this length, we have only been able to consider a few perspectives. We accept that many perspectives that readers may regard as vital are absent. If that is the case for you personally, we would love to hear from and learn from you (although we cannot promise to publish your perspective). Do consider reading chapters from unfamiliar perspectives with an open mind, as they may be those that precisely offer you the richest reflection on the challenges you face in your own context.

We cannot too strongly emphasise that coproduction should not become an end in itself. We suggest that two things matter most: social inclusion and agency. People living with human distress or mental health problems have as much right to enjoy the benefits of society as anyone else. Government (or other) resources should serve that end, in such a way that furthers their wellbeing alongside that of others. As to agency (or choice), many people may prefer alternatives to mainstream mental health services, and coproduction should support them where their choices are reasonable (obviously, vested interests may resist this).

We have deliberately allowed authors to use their own definitions of coproduction, so long as it involved service users, carers and staff in partnership. As you read each chapter, do consider the authors' choices and what led them to make them. You may want to revise your preferred definition or choose another. You may also recognise the diversity of terms used to describe participants in coproduction.

Although we argue that coproduction is ethically necessary and potentially more effective economically, we invite you to evaluate the debate. Coproducing every decision is quite unnecessary, although, as Chambers and colleagues (2014) illustrate in the case of emergency detentions, we can with imagination coproduce more than might be immediately obvious.

Were coproduction to become mainstream, we would need to avoid it turning into another set of targets decided in advance by the experts by profession. Yet, if it is primarily about relationships, how do we ensure its progress? Tritter and McCallum (2006) challenge its measurability, and it may be that coproduction itself can free us from our obsession with measuring everything (Raffay, 2016).

References

Arnstein, S. (1969). A ladder of citizen participation. *Journal of the American Institute of Planners, 35*, 216–224.

Barker, P.J. (2003). The tidal model: Psychiatric colonization, recovery and the paradigm shift in mental health care. *International Journal of Mental Health Nursing, 12*, 96–102.

Baxter, H., Mugglestone, M. & Maher, L. (2010). *The experience-based design approach: Concepts and case studies.* NHS Institute for Innovation and Improvement.

Chambers, M., Gallagher, A., Borschmann, R., Gillard, S., Turner, K. & Kantaris, X. (2014). The experiences of detained mental health service users: Issues of dignity in care. *BMC Medical Ethics, 1*, 1–8.

Church, K. & Reville, D. (1989). User involvement in the mental health field in Canada. *Canada's Mental Health, 37*, 22–25.

Cooke, A. (Ed.). (2014). *Understanding psychosis and schizophrenia: Why people sometimes hear voices, believe things that others find strange, or appear out of touch with reality, and what can help.* British Psychological Society.

Department of Health. (2006). *Our health, our care, our say: A new direction for community services.* The Stationery Office.

Department of Health and Social Care. (2015). *The NHS constitution: The NHS belongs to us all.* Department for Health and Social Care.

Forrest, S., Risk, I., Masters, H. & Brown, N. (2000). Mental health service user involvement in nurse education: Exploring the issues. *Journal of Psychiatric and Mental Health Nursing, 7*, 51–57.

Francis, R. (2013). *Report of the Mid-Staffordshire NHS Foundation Trust public inquiry: Executive summary.* The Stationery Office.

Horgan, Á. (2012). Review: Service user involvement in the evaluation of psycho-social intervention for self-harm: A systematic literature review. *Journal of Research in Nursing, 18*, 131–132.

Hubble, M., Duncan, B. & Miller, S. (1999). *The heart and soul of change: What works in therapy.* American Psychological Association.

Hui, A. & Stickley, T. (2007). Mental health policy and mental health service user perspectives on involvement: A discourse analysis. *Journal of Advanced Nursing, 59*, 416–426.

Kara, H. (2013). Mental health service user involvement in research: Where have we come from, where are we going? *Journal of Public Mental Health, 12*, 122–135.

Lencioni, P. (2002). *The five dysfunctions of a team: A leadership fable.* Wiley.

Mudhoni, C. (2014). *Service user involvement: Development of a communication strategy between service users and senior management in a healthcare voluntary organisation.* [Unpublished master's thesis.] Royal College of Surgeons in Ireland.

Oliver, K., Kothari, A. & Mays, N. (2019). The dark side of coproduction: Do the costs outweigh the benefits for health research? *Health Research Policy and Systems, 17*(33). https://doi.org/10.1186/s12961-019-0432-3

Os, J.V., Kenis, G. & Rutten, B. (2010). The environment and schizophrenia. *Nature, 48*, 203–212.

Pine II, B.J. (1999). *Mass customization: The new frontier in business competition.* Harvard Business Press.

Raffay, J. (2016). The Francis Report (2013): Neo-pharisaism in the NHS? *Health and Social Care Chaplaincy, 4*, 20–34.

Raffay, J. (2020). *The relationship between mental health services and faith communities: A co-produced grounded theory study.* [Doctoral thesis.] University of Durham.

Schizophrenia Commission. (2012). *The abandoned illness: A report from the Schizophrenia Commission.* Schizophrenia Commission.

Schön, D.A. (1984). *The reflective practitioner: How professionals think in action.* Basic Books.

Sedgwick, P. (1982). *Psycho politics.* Pluto Press.

Slay, J. & Stephens, L. (2013). *Co-production in mental health: A literature review.* New Economics Foundation.

Staniszewska, S., Mockford, C., Gibson, A., Herron-Marx, S. & Putz, R. (2012). Moving forward: Understanding the negative experiences and impacts of patient and public involvement in health service planning, development, and evaluation. In M. Barnes & P. Cotterell (Eds.), *Critical perspectives on user involvement* (pp.129–141). Policy Press.

Storm, M. & Edwards, A. (2013). Models of user involvement in the mental health context: Intentions and implementation challenges. *Psychiatric Quarterly, 84*, 313–327.

Survivors History Group. (2012). Survivors History Group takes a look at historians. In M. Barnes & P. Cotterell (Eds.), *Critical perspectives on user involvement* (pp.7–18). Policy Press.

Tritter, J. & McCallum, A. (2006). The snakes and ladders of user involvement: Moving beyond Arnstein. *Health Policy, 76*, 156–168.

Walsh, J., McSherry, W. & Kevern, P. (2013). The representation of service users' religious and spiritual concerns in care plans. *Journal of Public Mental Health, 12*, 153–164.

Section 1

Navigating coproduction:
Exploring the context of
coproduction in services

Navigating coproduction: Introduction

Julian Raffay and Pamela Fisher

In the film *Titanic* (Cameron, 1997), the salvage co-ordinator says of the ship's captain: 'Twenty-six years of experience working against him […] everything he knows is wrong.' Even as the ship was heading for the iceberg, its senior managers were calling for more speed. 'Crazy', you might think? Rather, outright 'madness'. Yet, as we look at the NHS, we see the very same psychology driving mental health services towards disaster.

We see the obsession with targets building the same head of steam that caused the Mid-Staffordshire scandal (Francis, 2013). Senior managers are calling for more speed, more output, more targets, while no one listens to the lookouts. We, the co-authors of the chapters in this section, feel very much like lookouts. We are making our voices heard because we see disaster on the horizon. We are sounding the alarm because we care about the passengers – and, indeed, about the crew. We care very much, which is why we are pleading for an immediate change of direction.

Our message is simple: we need to change course before it is too late. The 'broken and demoralised system' (Schizophrenia Commission, 2012, p.4) will break up if the NHS does not at the very least slow down and hear the people on deck. Just as the lookouts on the Titanic (the ship) had a vital role, so too do many service users and carers who, like us, are calling for services to take a different direction. This different direction is not one we can reach through mutiny. Please be assured, we have no plans to throw senior managers, psychiatrists, nurses and others of the NHS mental health workforce overboard. The genius of coproduction, at least according to Slay and Stephen's definition, is that it affirms everyone's contribution as 'vital' (Slay & Stephens, 2013, p.3).

From this perspective, senior managers, psychiatrists, nurses and similar are not our enemies – quite the opposite. They matter to us and we care about them. It is the system that is rubbish (although ruder words seem more appropriate). As in the film, *Titanic*, it is the system that is calling for more speed, that is threatening all our safety. That said, as human beings, we are sometimes prone to wait for change from above while failing to recognise our own agency. Coproduction should remind us that our everyday micro responses and behaviours can perpetuate and reinforce systems of inequality, or they can point towards something new.

Unlike the lookouts on the Titanic, our message is altogether more sophisticated, more nuanced. We are not simply hoping to avoid disaster; we intend to explore the way ahead. In doing so, we are looking to avoid quick fixes and simplistic solutions. It is not enough just to avoid the icebergs. We want to critically question the proposed approach and intended trajectory, in collaboration with others.

This is why we changed the title of this section from 'Successes in Coproduction' to 'Navigating Coproduction'. We changed tack (forgive the nautical pun), not because we could not find enough 'successes' but because we wanted to draw attention to coproduction's relational focus. Our experience is that many advocates of coproduction are calling for a quite different kind of service – one focused as much on relationships as on structures. We simply do not believe that the emotional deserts we have encountered on many psychiatric wards have so much as a cat's chance in hell of making people better. Our shout may sound shrill, but we feel that is appropriate. However, we absolutely have no desire to discourage so many excellent staff who work against the odds.[1]

We back our observations and personally painful experiences with Forrest and associates' stark finding that 'if a nurse cannot function at the "human" end of the continuum, there cannot be progress towards professional help' (Forrest et al., 2000, p.53). Their assertion might seem surprising in an organisation calling itself a *care* trust. Tragically, feeling cared for is a rare experience for service users and carers, not to mention staff. This became plain to me (JR) recently when a staff member at Mersey Care's Spirituality Lived Experience Advisory Panel expressed surprise at how much they had enjoyed the meeting, saying, 'It was amazing, it felt like people cared for and respected each other.' How strange!

The late Peter Gilbert, a professor (with lived experience), once asked: 'Why do we find it so hard to be and do human?' (personal communication,

---

1. To repeat, it is the system that we see as thwarting their best efforts and dehumanising service users, carers and staff alike.

2010). Coproduction is precisely about relationships – authentic relationships, in contrast with Kesey's 'combine' (2005). We reckon it is precisely because alternative forms of help and support, such as faith communities – at their best – offer warm, genuinely caring relationships that service users and carers often choose them ahead of mental health services (Raffay, 2020).

We can draw on our experiences of shopping, travelling by train or eating out to connect with that sense of being either genuinely cared for or treated as a commodity. For those who have been neglected, mistreated, abused or just marginalised by poverty, that will be even more the case. If we think we can pull the wool over people's eyes, we are the fools, not them.

I (JR) recall the spontaneous care I received after a head injury. A nurse in Accident and Emergency hugged me, briefly holding the injured side of my face to herself, and fetched me some sandwiches. She knew me. Her response was heartfelt, sincere and very much at 'the human end of the continuum'. A more considered approach probably would not have hugged me, or might have hugged my non-injured side (after carefully weighing up the risk of infection), and would undoubtedly have found a way to invoice me for the sandwiches! Her gesture brought light in my dark place. Do not misunderstand me; I was also grateful for the medical interventions I later received!

When we ask service users and carers what helped them recover, we typically find hugely different answers from those the clinicians are obliged to give. Before we conclude they are biased, it may be that, as Forrest and colleagues suggest, the best outcomes are likely to result from considering everyone's 'vital' contribution – through coproduction. As you read the chapters in this section (and throughout the book), we invite you to consider both the scientific and the human arguments being advanced.

Although each sheds its own light, you may want to ask what is common to all, and what unique aspects may be relevant to your own concerns. Gemma Stacey, Anne Felton and colleagues' ward round supplies an excellent opportunity to recognise what coproduction offers over and above involvement. Their chapter introduces the important question of whether coproduction is primarily about processes or outcomes. Coproduction, as Kris Southby, Frank Keating and Stephen Joseph write so compellingly in the chapter that follows, offers us all a way forward and may help us recognise our impact on other minority groups. Towards the end of their chapter, they introduce the important matter of agency – an area where coproduction really comes into its own.

Coercion and power are the main concerns of the next chapter, by Mark Chandley and AB. We faced huge ethical challenges around AB, the co-author with lived experience in high-secure services. We had to balance his author's rights with the potential political storm we risked were we to disclose his identity (or act in such a way that it could be inferred). So, in came paternalism and out went agency. These are hardly the kind of choices a coproduction team wishes to address, but we felt compelled to use the principles of informed consent and best interests. We would of course support his right to be identified as author on his return to the community. We accept that many may consider we failed him.

High-security services' extreme nature gives us insights into the more day-to-day coercive practices of mental health wards. Coproduction can bring a measure of honesty to both sides of those forced to live alongside each other in the same restrictive premises. In being honest, we accept that victims of violent crime may quite understandably find Mark and AB's text unsettling. As editors, we neither condone nor collude with alleged or actual offences. However, we fully support Mark and AB's desire for an approach that fosters genuinely transformative therapeutic outcomes and minimises purposeless human warehousing.

In this section's final chapter, Elaine Harrison artfully sets out a story of her life in 15 numbered scenes and a postscript. These vignettes, reminiscent of a film storyboard, serve not only as a personal history but also as a carefully choreographed account of instances that can be understood as coproduction. It is a life story presented as moral lesson in coproduction. Setbacks are offset by developments and opportunities that are shaped by co-operation, whether planned or fortuitous. The self-conscious sub-title of the chapter – 'a non-academic perspective' – helps to situate the everyday interpretations and examples of 'coproduction' here as a resource. What should that word mean? Whose perspectives on that question should matter? Academic or non-academic? Elaine's chapter helps remind us of the challenge that, just as much as mental healthcare, the very notion of coproduction should be coproduced.

We conclude our introduction by referring to Kara's (2013, p.131) concept of 'mutable' identities. Service users, carers and staff are not discrete groups, only roles. Keyes' (2002) notion of a mental health continuum understands wellbeing as a scale we all move up and down. Those who get locked up in the Titanic's steerage class are commonly those who suffer 'multiple overwhelmings' (Ford, 2012, pp.xvi-xvii), who are least understood by the dominant social order. Health inequalities reflect social inequalities and coproduction helps redress the balance.

References

Cameron, J. (Dir.). (1997). *Titanic*. [Film.] 20th Century Fox.

Ford, D. (2012). *The shape of living: Spiritual directions for everyday life*. Canterbury Press.

Forrest, S., Risk, I., Masters, H. & Brown, N. (2000). Mental health service user involvement in nurse education: Exploring the issues. *Journal of Psychiatric and Mental Health Nursing, 7*, 51–57.

Francis, R. (2013). *Report of the Mid-Staffordshire NHS Foundation Trust public inquiry: Executive summary*. The Stationery Office.

Kara, H. (2013). Mental health service user involvement in research: Where have we come from, where are we going? *Journal of Public Mental Health, 12*, 122–135.

Kesey, K. (2005). *One flew over the cuckoo's nest: A novel*. Penguin.

Keyes, C. (2002). The mental health continuum: From languishing to flourishing in life. *Journal of Health and Social Behaviour, 43*, 207–222.

Raffay, J. (2020). *The relationship between mental health services and faith communities: A co-produced grounded theory study*. [Doctoral thesis.] University of Durham.

Schizophrenia Commission (2012). *The abandoned illness: A report from the Schizophrenia Commission: Main report*. Schizophrenia Commission.

Slay, J. & Stephens, L. (2013). Co-production in mental health: A literature review. New Economics Foundation.

Chapter 1

Towards the ideal ward round: A coproduced service improvement project

Gemma Stacey, Anne Felton, involvement volunteers and members of the Ideal Ward Round Steering Group

This chapter explores the journey of a coproduced service improvement project that took place in a large mental health trust in the East Midlands, in England. The project was conceived by service user and carer volunteers. It focused on improving the experience of formal decision-making forums for people using and working in inpatient mental health services. These are often known as 'ward rounds'. To provide the context, we outline the coproduced process of the project, identifying key stages of its development and implementation. This is followed by a description of the journey, informed by the perspectives of those involved. This exploration is illuminated by extracts from discussions that captured reflections of meaningful and memorable events throughout the life of the project. The chapter concludes with a discussion of the role that power and influence have played at various points throughout the coproduced project. It will critically consider what that means for the concept of coproduction within a large statutory organisation.

Background

In the context of recovery-orientated care, shared decision-making is promoted as a valued approach that recognises service users' expertise and recognises their right to have a say in their treatment. Shared decision-making in acute inpatient mental health settings is complex, with constraining influences from institutional practices, staff groups and service user capacity (Stacey et al., 2015). Enabling service users to have choice and influence in decision-making remains a guiding principle, even when their capabilities may be impaired (Department of Health, 2015). The most common forum for decision-making in acute mental health environments is the ward round. Ward rounds have been acknowledged as important forums for information sharing. They are more helpful when service users have a good relationship with staff (Cappleman et al., 2015; Staniszewska et al., 2019). Yet, more commonly, ward rounds are perceived as an anxiety-provoking experience for service users in which they feel subject to staff power, with limited opportunity to exert influence (Cappleman et al., 2015). Psychiatrists, carers, nurses and other mental health professionals have also highlighted the ward round as problematic and recognise the challenges it can pose for service users to have their voices heard (Stacey et al., 2016).

This coproduced service development project, which would become known as the Ideal Ward Round (IWR) project, was initiated in 2014. Membership of the project group included:

- volunteers in the Involvement Centre[1] of a large NHS trust primarily providing mental healthcare services, who had used or cared for someone who had used the service and had experience of attending ward rounds
- the trust's Involvement and Experience Lead
- a group of academics and clinicians, known as the Critical Values-Based Practice Network, who had conducted research into shared decision-making in inpatient mental healthcare. They identified the ward round as the central decision-making structure that was viewed by all stakeholders as not fit for purpose (Stacey et al., 2016)
- an advocate with significant experience of the challenges associated with the ward round structure in terms of enabling the voice of the service user to be heard within this setting.

The idea for the IWR project was born from a shared motivation and commitment of these groups and individuals to change entrenched, routine practice. They began from a consensus that the current ward round process was both distressing for people using the service and their families, and dysfunctional in terms of organisation, procedure and satisfactory outcomes.

---

1. The Involvement Centre is a venue where people can get involved in a variety of activities and opportunities to provide input into shaping services, or to work on personal development in a welcoming and supportive environment.

A steering group was formed that met monthly at the Involvement Centre and was chaired by the Involvement Centre manager. The group had complete oversight of the planning, development and implementation of the project. Crucially, the project was initiated by people with lived experience and driven by a common interest and desire for change. There were no external drivers, funding or strategic goals to dictate or limit the vision of the project.

In an effort to ensure the project was underpinned by an extensive range of views, the group designed a questionnaire and conducted focus groups with staff, people using the service, and their families. Questionnaires were taken to the wards by Involvement Centre volunteers, who helped service users to complete them. Coproduction was an important principle at all stages of the project. The questionnaires and focus group prompts were co-designed by the IWR steering group, and the group also analysed the data, both qualitative and quantitative. The results reflected the views of the IWR project group – that there were several problems with the ward round structure in acute care. The survey also revealed a broadly consistent view among service users, carers and staff regarding what these problems were. The findings generated 12 recommendations for improving ward rounds (see Table 1.1).

Table 1.1: The Ideal Ward Round recommendations

- A clearly defined and communicated purpose of the ward round relative to the overall inpatient experience.
- To 'declutter' the ward round and to recommend how issues such as treatment, Section 17 leave and discharge planning may be resolved outside the ward round.
- Consideration for issues of power imbalance that currently exist between patients and professionals, carers and professionals and professionals themselves, establishing practice of joint ownership of the ward round.
- Practical application of both shared decision-making and supported decision-making, with emphasis on maximising patient autonomy and reducing substitute decision-making by healthcare professionals.
- A model where each ward round has an agreed 'agenda' into which all parties input and that is circulated in good time to allow for preparation and follow-up.
- Clear processes for the preparation and follow-up of ward rounds, ensuring participants are well prepared, actions are agreed and monitoring of actions is effective.
- Demonstration of supportive, person-centred discharge planning from admission, with a focus on the individual's recovery.
- Guidance on the appropriate length/duration of the ward round that is reasonable and proportionate to its aims, the involvement of relevant parties and relevant staffing resources.
- Consideration of the physical environment of the ward round and recommendations for ensuring this is welcoming and open and minimises anxiety and intimidation.

- A defined limit on the numbers who attend ward rounds to ensure that significantly fewer people attend than is current practice, with clear rationale and service user agreement for attendance.
- Particular attention to communication with and involvement of carers, and the potential barriers to this (e.g. confidentiality).
- A process for management, auditing and evaluation of ward rounds that allows measurement of patient, carer and professional satisfaction, continual improvement in practice and benchmarking standards.

The project then moved into the implementation phase. Three wards were identified as pilot sites across the geographical spread of the organisation to trial some or all of the recommendations. Staff members of the steering group and Involvement Centre volunteers met with the ward clinical leads and a baseline audit was conducted. This included both a self-audit by ward staff and questionnaires distributed by the IWR steering group. It was repeated at three- and six-month intervals. Alongside, the trust provided funding to collaboratively develop open-access, reusable educational resources to support staff in implementing the recommendations and link them to wider theory and policy.

The implementation was challenging. During this time, the steering group continued to meet to review and guide the process. This included providing strategic and organisational support to ensure impact at a ward level. The IWR group organised a launch event attended by the trust's general manager, clinical director, executive medical director, head of quality improvement, ward managers, service managers and consultants to facilitate organisational commitment to implementation. The project was adopted by the trust's quality improvement team. The clinical director met with the group to draft guidelines for the ward round to be included in the trust's adult mental health safe and timely discharge policy. The IWR steering group continues to meet bimonthly to monitor and support the implementation of the recommendations across the trust's adult mental health services.

The following account is intended to offer an insight into the experience of engagement in the IWR project from a range of perspectives. Using the analogy of a journey, it shows what has facilitated and challenged this process and how the group's work has been underpinned by coproduction throughout. The quotes are taken from two facilitated reflective discussions with IWR group members and illuminate some of the central themes of the experience.

A shared desire to reach the destination

The IWR group was built on a collective desire to improve the experience of ward rounds for people using mental health services. Consequently, each meeting and activity was working towards a shared aim. Despite the individual members having varied motivations to be involved and varied roles within the organisation, this shared and single agenda appeared to create a level of cohesiveness and motivation that would prove to be invaluable to the process. The following extracts demonstrate some of these varied motivations:

> ... the patients kept telling me about ward rounds for many years and I could understand and put myself in the same position. I wouldn't like to go into somewhere and have half a dozen people looking at me. I would freeze and I'd just think to myself, 'I want to get out of here.' I wouldn't tell you anything. I'd just want to go. And so, I thought that can't be right, there must be another way around it, but that's where it has come from over the years. (Volunteer)

> You just realise how challenging the environment is and how locked it feels and how difficult it feels to have therapeutic, positive conversations, particularly when people's liberties are restricted and so many constraints. And anything that could make that a bit better so that you could push up the service user and family voice within that. Anything that helps, even a little bit would be seen as positive. (Psychologist)

> Initially as a ward manager, you have lots of plates and you're spinning [them] all the time and lots of people [are] needing pieces of you but this sort of thing has a value, but as a person as well, it's helping the patients. It's helping the people that we're serving. It is helping the people and that's what we're here to do. (Ward manager)

These extracts illustrate the shared value base held by members of the IWR group. This was underpinned by a recognition of the lack of power and influence the person using mental health services has within the ward round structure. They reflect a desire to enable the voice of the person to be actively heard and inherently influential in the decision-making process. While this represents a complex notion in relation to human rights, law and professional accountability, in essence it was seen as a simple and tangible task that few people within the organisation would disagree with:

> I've had this idea, what would it – what would the model look like for a ward round that was perfect? And it's a really easy idea. It's a really simple idea. We've discovered that actually it is a very complex thing to do but, as an idea, it's something you can understand within two minutes. You can say exactly what it is. And that part of it really chimed because I

thought, this is a thing that I understand, and we can create the story of this and people will understand what we're trying to do. So that, I think, that was the motivation for it. I didn't know what it would be, but I could see an end point, which was, we are going to create a model for a ward round that will be better for service users and carers. And I could see that that's what we're going to do. (Involvement Centre manager)

A consistent and facilitative navigator

When considering what has enabled the group process underpinning the IWR project, there was a consensus around the value of a consistent person who could facilitate the project. In our case, this was the Involvement Centre manager, who was employed by the trust to promote public engagement in the development and monitoring of the trust's activities. On a superficial level, this involved the complex co-ordination and implementation of the project (e.g. room bookings, scheduling diaries, recording meetings and admin support), which other members of the group had not been given authority by the trust to do. However, the following quotes demonstrate that the manager's skilled and inclusive approach was highly influential to the way the group worked towards their goal.

> Linking both with people, the volunteers, people coming through the Involvement Centre, and also sitting in lots of meetings and linking with the trust. But this kind of interface bridge between the group which is the service users and carers that use our services and come in and the organisation that provides that, and having that daily connection between the two, I think, was an ideal position to be there. So, I think there's something about the role. (Volunteer)

> You listen to what we say, you don't just hear what we say. You just listen and, like you said, if somebody did come up with a really wacky idea, you wouldn't make that person feel like we shouldn't have said that. It doesn't matter what we've said, but I feel it's nothing at all what we've said, but you've taken account of what we have said, and you might have just gone, 'So I actually don't agree with you.' But you've never given me the impression that you're thinking, 'She's at it again.' You probably did, but you never gave away yourself. (Volunteer)

These extracts show how the qualities, principles and organisational position of this individual facilitated the progress of the project. It was clear, throughout the reflective discussions, that trust and sincerity were key to the relationships that enabled the group to work in a collaborative manner. It appears that the Involvement Centre manager modelled these attributes in his approach to leading the project, which influenced the relational practices within the group.

A willingness to pick up friends along the way

The IWR group was initially open to all volunteers and staff interested in the agenda. However, over time, a collective decision was made to have a stable membership, to enable progress and ensure contributors were aware of the historical context of the group's activity.

> I can think of probably three or four times when people came in that – I don't know if they've ever had an intention of staying with a group or not. I wasn't really quite clear, but they weren't necessarily helpful influences. There have been other people that came along for one or two meetings that were kind of very dogmatic. And that's annoying for me because I was thinking, 'You've just arrived.' (Volunteer)

Conversely, the group also acknowledged where they would require the support and expertise of external people who offered both knowledge and organisational influence. An example of this was when conducting the thematic analysis of interview and focus group data. The group invited a qualitative researcher with experience of collaborative approaches to data analysis.

The group also described an active approach to co-opting friends with influence. This included members of the senior leadership team within the trust who were viewed as having a shared motivation and a level of organisational influence that would support the potential of the project to have influence. These relationships became increasingly important as the project progressed.

A naïve optimism that we've reached our destination

The IWR group members reflected on some significant events that were memorable to them as individuals. The events related to tasks undertaken as part of the project, which they approached with a seemingly naïve optimism. This appeared to be underpinned by a faith in the group's collective ability to navigate these challenges and willingness to commit the time it would take. One example was the development of the reusable learning object (RLO), which aimed to engage staff in an online learning activity to enable their understanding of the importance of the IWR recommendations.[2]

---

2. The RLO is an open access online learning resource that was developed by the IWR group for the purpose of informing and engaging staff in the 12 recommendations. It is available at www.nottingham.ac.uk/helmopen/rlos/mentalhealth/ward-round

> When we watched the first clip of – it was the actor, wasn't it? Walking, getting up from bed and walking through the corridors and then came into the room. And it was just really, really powerful, I thought, which shocked me actually because I'm used to lots of online learning for the trust, and doing all that. But it really, really kind of captured, I thought, the essence of what it must feel like to be on a ward and I was really impressed with it, actually. I thought the group's done something really good. But again, that took years, just the staying power, and that's why I think what the group has had is staying power, which has been really important. (Psychologist)

Another significant event related to working with an acute inpatient ward to implement the recommendations. Members of the IWR group, including the volunteers and a ward manager, described rearranging the room where the ward round was conducted. They removed the tables and arranged the chairs in a small circle, to try to make the environment less formal and intimidating for the service user. However, the next people to use the room just moved the furniture back to its original arrangement, which symbolised the ingrained culture the group was attempting to challenge.

> We said about potentially changing it – should we do it, should we change it, what should we do? And everyone was like, yes that's good. And we got the tables out. We moved the tables out to the side. We had the chairs in a nice circular position. And we said, rather than people sitting here with their backs to the door and their backs to the people who are typing, we would seat them there, so they could see everybody in the room. And then we wouldn't have tables, because people can put laptops on their knees. Brilliant. We looked at it all. We took a photo of it and we said 'Brilliant, let's leave it like this. Let's see what happens.' I remember I went out and told the staff, leave the room like that because the review was the next day. I went to a meeting and came out at lunchtime, walked into the review room and everything was back to normal. The tables were moved back in the middle of the room. There were laptops on the tables, and it felt so frustrating. And so, the following day, I went to the consultant and said, 'What happened to the room?' And he said, not in any kind of negative way, 'Whoever did it left the room the other way, so we just put it back to how it normally is.' (Ward manager)

> That was a really vivid memory for me, because it was kind of symbolic. It was so kind of evocative of the nub of the challenge of trying to work

with a system to make a change against huge amounts of powerful forces, not just at that time and that place, but throughout kind of like the history of mental health and the doctor–patient relationship and the doctor–nurse relationship and the Mental Health Act. It kind of seemed to be crystallised, almost, and we've gone in and made what you kind of think was a relatively benign, innocuous change. (Psychologist)

In response to this event and lack of progress, some professional members of the IWR group began to lose faith in the ability of the group to influence change:

But ultimately, we're still in the position where the ward rounds are not that different and so to keep going and keep going, and I think we were all – I certainly was – kind of pretty close to saying – you throw your hands up and say, 'What more power do we have?' (Psychologist)

This included the Involvement Centre manager, who said he wanted to close down the project and acknowledge the limits of the group's power, as its members were only volunteers. It was suggested that the constraints in terms of consistent staffing, clinical priorities and ingrained institutional practices represented significant blocks to culture change from the bottom up. Despite this, the volunteers were unwilling to accept defeat until their motivation to improve the experience of ward rounds had been realised. This was based on a trust in the collective ability of the group to find a way to overcome these challenges and an inherent faith in the Involvement Centre manager to enable this to happen.

'Oh, we've done this thing. Let's be pleased with this thing and then close it down because we just didn't know what to do.' I think there's something really interesting about me not having control of that, about it not actually being my decision to make and, as a group, we've always made decisions going forward together. So actually, it's not any individual's decision. And there's something interesting that you'd say that about the responsibility for people outside of this group that motivates you, and in some respect, that's why it has continued, isn't it? Has it just been about these people? Have there been other staff members that have come in? On the journey of the project itself, there's been a lot of different staff members that have come through the group and a lot of different people as well, and that, in some ways, has strengthened it. Because you can't shut it down without anyone noticing. You have a responsibility to continue it for all those people that have heard the story a little bit. (Involvement Centre manager)

Agreeing when the destination has been reached

This event demonstrates the differing views of the professionals and volunteers as to the point at which the destination had been reached. Despite his reservations, the Involvement Centre manager responded positively to the volunteers' wishes to continue, and the decision was made to invest the group's energies in gaining the support and sponsorship of senior leaders within the trust. The group viewed this as a constructive action that re-energised their hope for positive change:

> We thought, 'Yeah, we're going somewhere again,' and I felt really elated at that time. Well, I felt exactly the same. What have we been doing all this time? But we understood where you were coming from because it wasn't going anywhere. It was in our best interest. But then I thought, 'If it's not going anywhere and we're pushing it, it needs to be pushed from upstairs and somebody up there saying "Well, I agree with this and this is what we're going to do".' (Volunteer)

The change in approach was achieved by drawing on existing relationships with allies with influence and using their power within the organisation to instil the recommendations in policy and quality monitoring. This was facilitated by the executive medical director, who initiated a launch event and insisted on clinical staff coming along, including professional groups who are notoriously hard to engage due to lack of interest or difficulty being released from clinical duties.

> It was really a significant turn. I was utterly amazed at how many people came off the wards. Getting one member of staff released is incredibly difficult. So, to have that many people here was incredible – really, much more than I thought, I have to say. (Psychologist)

For the IWR group, this was the point in the journey where they agreed that they had reached their destination. It represented a stage in the voyage where the power to influence had been handed over to senior leaders within the organisation and the group was depending on them to ensure the changes were implemented. The group reflected their feelings towards this process with a sense of pride, but also resolve. Their efforts to influence the organisation from the bottom up had been met with significant barriers. This led them to conclude that there was a point where coproduction ended and the organisation needed to take ownership and use its power and influence to initiate and embed the change.

> It felt as though we were handing the baton over a bit, to me anyway. And at least those people wanted to make something happen. What happens eventually, who knows? It felt like they wanted to do it. (Volunteer)

Coproduction in action

Coproduction involves groups of people working together as equals in decision-making while valuing each other's perspectives (Springham & Robert, 2015). The process we have described demonstrates that our practice has held coproduction at its heart. Several of the factors perceived as facilitating this process resonate with the findings from research on the factors that facilitate coproduction within large statutory organisations. Of relevance was the shared commitment to the project outcomes and the belief that coproduction was the right way to achieve this. Clark (2015) suggests this shared motivation is the catalyst for service users and professionals to work together, mediating the influence of professional hierarchies and traditional power dynamics. The volunteers very clearly recognised the Involvement Centre manager (our navigator) as facilitating the establishment of the flexible and responsive interpersonal relationships that Palumbo (2016) suggests will enable supportive conditions and promote reciprocity and engagement for the purposes of coproduction.

The IWR project grew out of a safe and collaborative space (the Involvement Centre). This environment and the relational practices it enabled resonate with Needham (2008), who advocates the benefits of meeting in neutral spaces (i.e. outside the ward or treatment centre), where service users and providers/professionals can collaborate to share experiences and agree on service improvements.

Carr (2016) maintains that the first phase of coproduction that transforms services and communities can be collaborative but may also be confrontational, because of the need to challenge institutional rules and expose unhelpful cultural norms. This is particularly relevant to the setting of the IWR project, as inpatient mental health wards are dominated by the bio-medical model, which is challenged through the practice of coproduction (Palumbo, 2016).

The IWR group assumed their work would pave the way for service redesign/improvement. However, in reality, the group's attempt to implement the IWR recommendations had limited impact on practice. Implementation had to be handed back to the hierarchy of the organisation when embedded institutional cultures proved too challenging for the group to overcome.

However, this may also reflect some of the limitations of the parties involved in the IWR steering group, which lacked representation from staff working in acute inpatient care. The danger in this is that attempts to change ward rounds are viewed as top-down rather than bottom-up initiatives, resulting in opposition to attempts to change routine practice on the wards (Fiddler et al., 2010).

The group acknowledged that shared vision and consensus are central to collaborative approaches but that conflict is also a significant feature of coproduction and can have the power to transform. Another limitation may have been lack of challenge and critical dialogue within the group.

Conclusion

The ambition and commitment of the IWR group cannot be faulted. Coproduction was both the motivation for the service improvement and the mechanism adopted to achieve it. This influenced process and decisions at each phase, including development of the ideas, collection of data, interpretation and planning of implementation. What has become clear to us it that good coproductive processes and values are not enough to make sustainable changes to ingrained cultural practice. What has been achieved are some ripples in the ocean and what is needed is a wave to carry our vision forward.

References

Cappleman, R., Bamford, Z., Dixon, C. & Thomas, H. (2015). Experiences of ward rounds among in-patients on an acute mental health ward: A qualitative exploration. *BJPsych Bulletin, 39*(5), 233–236.

Carr, S. (2016). *Position paper: Are mainstream mental health services ready to progress transformative coproduction?* National Development Team for Social Inclusion.

Clark, M. (2015). Coproduction in mental health care. *The Mental Health Review, 20*(4), 213–219.

Department of Health. (2015). *Mental Health Act: Code of practice*. The Stationery Office. https://assets.publishing.service.gov.uk/government/uploads/system/uploads/attachment_data/file/435512/MHA_Code_of_Practice.PDF

Fiddler, M., Borglin, G., Galloway, A., Jackson, C., McGowan, L. & Lovell, K. (2010). Once-a-week psychiatric ward round or daily inpatient team meeting? A multidisciplinary mental health team's experience of new ways of working. *International Journal of Mental Health Nursing, 19*(2), 119–127.

Needham, C. (2008). Realising the potential of co-production: Negotiating improvements in public services. *Social Policy and Society, 7*(2), 221–231.

Palumbo R. (2016). Contextualising coproduction of health care: A systematic literature review. *International Journal of Public Sector Management, 29*(1), 72–90.

Springham, N. & Robert, G. (2015). Experience based co-design reduces formal complaints on an acute mental health ward. *BMJ Open Quality, 4*(1).

Stacey, G., Felton, A., Houghton, P., Hui, A., Morgan, A., Shutt, J., Diamond, B., Willis, M. & Stickley, T. (2015). Informed, involved and influential: The 3 I's model of shared decision making in mental health care. *Mental Health Practice, 19*(4), 31–35.

Stacey, G., Felton, A., Morgan, A., Stickley, T., Willis, M., Diamond, B., Houghton, P., Johnson, B. & Dumenya, J. (2016). A critical narrative analysis of shared decision-making in acute inpatient mental health care. *Journal of Interprofessional Care, 30*(1), 35–41.

Staniszewska, S., Mockford, C., Chadburn, G., Fenton, S.J., Bhui, K., Larkin, M., Newton, E., Crepaz-Keay, D., Griffiths, F. & Weich, S. (2019). Experiences of in-patient mental health services: Systematic review. *The British Journal of Psychiatry, 214*(6), 329–338.

Chapter 2

Mental health recovery through coproduction: African and Caribbean men's experiences in the United Kingdom

Kris Southby, Frank Keating and Stephen Joseph

In this chapter, we explore the role of coproduction in the mental health recovery of men of African and Caribbean heritage ('Black men') in the UK. We draw on our own research into socially orientated approaches to recovery for Black men in London and Leeds, and on the wider literature. The chapter adopts a broad understanding of coproduction. In addition to commonly held notions of coproduction being about citizens and professionals sharing power to plan and deliver support together (Slay & Stephens, 2013), we suggest that, to facilitate mental health recovery for Black men in the UK, coproduction also needs to include citizens sharing power with other citizens. We argue that Black men engaging in more coproductive practices with peers, family, friends and wider communities, as well as professionals, provides them with opportunities to find safety, experience trusting relationships, (re)establish productive social identities and exert agency, all of which form the basis of their recovery.

Black men and mental health in the UK

Racial disparities in mental health prevalence and services in the UK are long-standing and well documented (Sainsbury Centre for Mental Health, 2006). Initiatives designed to reduce these inequalities have been introduced by successive governments – sadly, with little effect. The Delivering Race

Equality programme (Department of Health, 2005), for example, was launched in 2005 with a specific aim to improve mental healthcare and treatment for Black, Asian and minoritised ethnic communities in England. Despite some positive outcomes, nearly 15 years after its introduction, the situation for these communities has not significantly improved.

The Care Quality Commission (2013) has shown persisting inequalities in mental health for people from across Black, Asian and minoritised ethnic communities, and particularly those with African and Caribbean heritage. Black men, specifically, are over-represented in the mental health system, report inferior experiences and achieve poorer outcomes. The Chief Medical Officer's most recent report on mental health (Davies, 2014) describes how these men are more likely to be given a diagnosis of schizophrenia; are more likely to be admitted to hospital via police intervention; have higher rates of detention under the Mental Health Act; are more likely to receive the harsher kind of treatments, such as control and restraint; are more likely to be held in seclusion and on locked wards, and are less likely to be offered socially orientated interventions. Mental health is not divorced from social context, and Black men in the UK also experience persistent inequalities in social domains such as poverty and unemployment, which exert a significant effect on both physical and mental health (Cabinet Office, 2017).

Our study

We were funded by the National Institute of Health Research's School for Social Care Research (NIHR-SSCR) to investigate to what extent socially orientated approaches to recovery can better support Black men in the UK to break out of the stalled 'cycle of recovery'. The work took place between 2016 and 2018 in London and Leeds.

We carried out in-depth interviews with 30 Black men, who were at different points in their recovery journey, about their experiences of mental health recovery. We asked the men to nominate someone who they felt had supported them in an informal capacity during their recovery (e.g. family, friend, church leader, work colleague) and someone from a statutory service who they felt had provided them with more formal support. We interviewed 15 of these informal 'supporters' and 14 formal service 'providers' through this route. Some of the men were unwilling to nominate a formal service provider because they felt their recovery journey was personal and that they had received little or no support from mental health professionals.

Following completion of all the interviews, we held co-creation events in London and Leeds for the men we had interviewed to reflect on the emergent themes from the interviews and what they thought should be done to support the mental health recovery of Black men in the UK in the future. Many of the men appreciated the opportunity to engage with their peers in this way and found the experience very therapeutic. We also held a symposium in London to discuss emergent findings with health and social care professionals. We used interpretative phenomenological analysis (IPA) to analyse the data gathered from the interviews, co-creation events and symposium. The analysis looked for personal significance, important relationships and significant events, and how these contribute to, support or otherwise affect recovery.

For the men we spoke to, recovery was experienced as a journey that was intrinsically tied to both their mental health experiences and broader life histories. They understood their mental health recovery as the latest struggle in lives characterised by ongoing adversity inherent to being a Black man in the UK.

Family was both a source of strength and a challenge across the life course for these men. Families provided emotional, pastoral and practical support and a place of safety, but family dysfunction and breakdown were traumatising. Separation, often tied to migration, was a consistent theme. Living in a racialised society was another persistent issue for the men. As well as overt racism, the men commonly felt stigmatised and 'othered' in society. Many of the men felt they lacked positive role models and were generally expected to adhere to hegemonic masculine norms: to be seen as strong, tough and not vulnerable, as a provider and not dependent on others.

The men attributed their mental ill health to traumatic early life experiences, substance misuse, supernatural events and genetics. Although the meaning of recovery was deeply personal for each of them, there was a consensus that recovery is more holistic than a reduction in clinical measures. Common features included psychological and physical healing, social inclusion and living a 'normal life', control and agency, positive social identity, and aspirations for the future.

The men typically had given little thought to 'mental health' prior to their own experiences. For most of the men, their experience of mental ill health involved an accumulation of issues until they could no longer cope and displayed some unexpected or erratic behaviour that drew the attention of others, including the police. This is what Brownhill and colleagues (2005) refer to as a 'big build'. The men generally did not understand what they were going through, when to seek help or who they were seeing during the care process.

The mental healthcare the men received from statutory services was experienced as extremely depersonalised. Men felt they did not receive treatment and care that was tailored to them or culturally appropriate. Services were perceived as outcome focused (e.g. compliance with medication, symptom reduction), and offering very little space for them to explore what was important to them in their recovery. They regarded what they perceived as the overly medicalised treatment and care they received from statutory services as not helping them address the challenges they faced.

Robinson and colleagues (2011) suggest that Black men in the UK are likely to find themselves in a 'stalled cycle of recovery', in which they struggle to recover once they come into contact with statutory mental health services. This is due to a gendered reluctance to seek help, overlaid with a fear of services, negative perceptions of Black men within services as 'big, Black, and angry', poor quality and coercive treatment from services, and a worsening of mental health. These factors occur in a cyclical fashion to prevent mental health recovery. Positive support for the men in our study generally came from outside the statutory services, in the community. They found strength in the informal support of their peers and in the opportunities provided by community-based, third-sector organisations to socialise, engage in leisure activities and express themselves.

A model of mental health recovery for Black men in the UK

From our research, we concluded that mental health recovery for Black men in the UK is about them (re)gaining capability across four interconnected life domains: safe spaces, agency, identity and relationships (Figure 2.1). We say '(re)gaining' in recognition that some men may be acquiring something entirely new within these domains, while others may be rebuilding what was lost during their mental health journey. Our model is reflective of the idea that biological, social and institutional factors contribute to one's physical and mental health independently, interactively and cumulatively across the life course (Kuh & Hardy, 2002).

Safe spaces

The lives of many Black men in recovery in the UK are shaped by historical and ongoing personal, social, emotional and physical threats and challenges. These may be both perceived and actual. Black men therefore need spaces that are 'safe' to enable them to acquire a positive sense of self, form supportive relationships and regain the agency that is central to recovery. To the men we spoke to, 'safety' represented the absence of external physical and emotional violence or abuse, whether perceived or actual. Feeling 'safe' also manifested in terms of the relationships they had with other people; safe relationships were those built on trust and mutual understanding. Having a similar or common history, culture, beliefs and values built on lived experience played a significant role in the men feeling understood. Three broad areas were described around which the men felt a sense of mutual understanding: ethnicity, mental health experience and gender. These factors do not occur in isolation but overlap and

Figure 2.1: The four interconnected domains of mental health recovery for African and Caribbean men

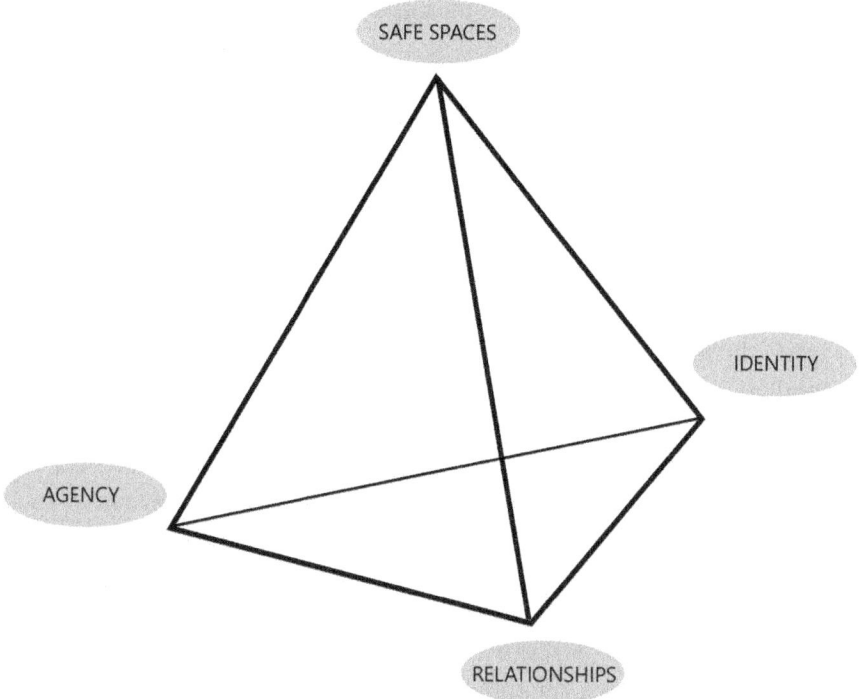

interact in a dynamic fashion to produce a hierarchy in which the safest spaces are those where shared lived experience is maximised.

Statutory mental health services were generally characterised as highly unsafe spaces as they lacked a sense of cultural consideration and gendered awareness and were perceived as depersonalised. These men did not want to speak freely with care providers for fear that their words would, at best, be misunderstood and at worst be used against them to justify prolonged hospitalisation and/or treatment. They particularly lamented what they perceived as a breach of trust when what they said was shared as case notes with other professionals, despite being told it would be private.

By comparison, non-statutory, community-based and third-sector organisations were thought to offer a safer space for Black men in recovery. The significance of a shared cultural heritage was extensively highlighted in relation to the perceived 'safety' of community-based spaces. Community organisations that were designed to meet the cultural needs of people with African and Caribbean heritage were described as 'home' (London, triad 11, man), and fellow service users and staff as 'extended family' (London, triad 14, provider). In contrast to what was perceived as 'white' health and care services, community-based organisations were seen to provide a venue for Black men to connect with their culture, faith and people who shared their lived experiences. Institutions such as churches and mosques also provided cultural and social touchstones.

However, 'the community' is by no means a default safe space or a panacea to all the problems faced by Black men in recovery. A number of those we spoke to described feeling alienated and ostracised from social and family networks because of stigma surrounding mental health. Such stigma is then internalised by the men themselves.

Considering where Black men feel safe raises issues about the accessibility of mental healthcare for people who are not in an acute stage of illness. It suggests the urgent need to set up safe spaces where Black men can express mental pain without feeling judged. While community-based spaces, particularly those focused on the needs of people of African and Caribbean heritage, are helpful sources of social support for Black men in recovery, they risk perpetuating the stigma of mental health. To paraphrase one man we spoke to, he did not want to go to a day centre run by a third-sector organisation 'because they deal with mental health'.

Relationships

Strong and supportive relationships were identified as facilitating the recovery of Black men in the UK. The men we spoke to found both practical and emotional support in relationships that were 'authentic'. This meant relationships characterised by genuine care within a positive relationship, rather than support delivered by someone who was impersonal and detached. The men were generally critical of their relationships with health and social care organisations, which they felt followed predetermined scripts and did not allow for dialogue or for strategies to be coproduced. One participant explained, 'To the NHS you're just a number' (Leeds, triad 3, man). These men were additionally critical of the power imbalances inherent in their relationships with professionals that privileged professional knowledge over other forms of knowledge (e.g. expertise by experience) and shut down opportunities for Black men to focus on what was important to them.

The men we spoke to found strength in relationships with other Black men and especially with other Black men who themselves had experience of mental ill health. Men emphasised the sense of togetherness that came from being with other men who had been through similar experiences. Such trusting relationships offered these men a space to open up and express their thoughts and feelings. However, they also described being mistrustful of other people of African and Caribbean heritage who held traditional understandings of masculinity and equated mental distress with weakness. They tried to avoid such relationships that perpetuated the type of misrecognition and stigma found elsewhere in society. For example, one man told us how he felt more comfortable at a mental health support group made up of men from various ethnic backgrounds rather than with his Black friends, who he felt did not understand his mental health experience.

Our findings strongly support the role of peer support and men's support groups. Central to the process of recovery is that such relationships provide opportunities for conversation on a range of subjects, rather than focusing specifically on mental distress. Discussing issues relevant to social recovery, such as work and social activities, helps create a supportive environment, enabling an asset-based approach to recovery. The relationships that participants enjoy in men's groups and from informal networks and supporters appear central to their finding the kind of recognition associated with family and friendship relationships (Honneth, 2001). In addition, if men have opportunities to engage in meaningful activities through peer support groups and/or with other members of support groups, they can benefit from the recognition associated with achievement (usually associated with employment and/or public activities) (Honneth, 2001). Through being able to share a range of experiences and provide mutual help, participants are facilitated to function more fully across diverse areas of life.

Identity

Before their mental illness, the men we spoke to commonly felt an expectation to be a 'strong *Black man*': to display strength and resilience rather than express weakness, emotion or a need for help. This hegemonic masculine identity may have contributed, at least in part, to the mental health difficulties of some of them, causing isolation and a fear of betraying their vulnerability, while closing down possibilities for growth. At the same time, hegemonic masculinity was, for many, an armour that had been acquired to survive in the face of daily actual or perceived physical and emotional threats dating back to childhood. Many were terrified that opening up and sharing vulnerability could result in the collapse of precarious coping mechanisms and/or the venting of aggression that had been internalised through experiences of past trauma. Their mental health experience was felt as a major 'biographical disruption' (Bury, 2002) that included loss of employment and personal and social roles and a sense of isolation, which contributed to a loss of sense of self. The process of recovery involved developing a social identity that the men were satisfied with. For many Black men in recovery in the UK, the question is whether they should seek to return to a previous sense of self or look to something new.

Along their recovery journeys, many men were appearing to reposition their identities away from rugged individualism towards a more relational orientation and more flexible or inclusive masculinities. This is when men across their life course adopt practices that are associated with other marginalised identities (Bridges & Pascoe, 2014). Renegotiating one's identity necessitates significant courage, a journey that many of the men we spoke to had clearly embarked on by reflecting on their identities, including taken-for-granted masculinities previously core to their sense of self. This involved seeking out emotionally supportive relationships in place of relationships that may have shored up a previous sense of self based on traditional masculinity.

These men were finding the necessary support from other Black men to undergo self-transformation, mainly in the context of support groups, which appeared to provide the type of social environment that facilitates more open engagement with others. A potentially worthwhile dimension of men's groups tailored to the needs of Black men is that they may offer opportunities for rediscovering collective and cultural identities. As one participant pointed out, having a secure sense of self stems at least partly from a strong sense of shared culture.

Offering community appears to be central to the success of men's groups. Community does not solely involve interpersonal support but comprises an embodied experience of wellbeing related to the provision of emotional, social and practical guidance. It can be tailored to men's particular needs, including sometimes the celebration of culture – for example, through food. Participants sometimes associated their discovery of solidarity in recovery with traditional 'African values'. This tended to be accompanied by an awareness that there is a need to rebuild community.

Agency

Agency and control are about a person's ability to shape their lives and act on the world, rather than having a sense of always being 'done to' by others (Sullivan, 2016). It was felt that Black men in recovery could exert their agency in a variety of ways. On a personal level, being able to exert control over one's body and symptoms of mental ill health was seen as an expression of agency. Other areas were being in control of both the overall direction of their lives and of more prosaic, day-to-day decisions. These men particularly stressed the importance of controlling their housing as an indication of independence and, therefore, of recovery. They wanted a range of activities that provided a structure that supported their agency and creativity – opportunities to explore existing interests and develop new talents.

To promote recovery, more opportunities are needed that enable Black men to engage in activities that they find meaningful, invoking what Bologh (1990) has termed 'aesthetic rationality'. Aesthetic rationality refers to an appreciation and responsiveness to beauty. This does not refer to the normal meaning of beauty but rather to an appreciation and responsiveness to all activities that enhance physical, social and emotional wellbeing, such as socialising, being creative, gardening, listening to music, dancing and so forth. The types of activities associated with aesthetic rationality are often shared. What we draw from this is that, while the activities are meaningful in themselves, part of their value stems from the connections with others, based on mutual recognition that enables men to rediscover their sense of self-worth and individual agency.

Our experience would suggest that recovery is not about Black men enacting agency based on a model of 'rugged' individualism. Agency to support recovery was instead interpreted as striking a balance between independence and support and having the knowledge about where to find the most appropriate help. Such balance was not generally achieved within relationships with statutory mental health services. On the one hand, these Black men commonly viewed statutory services as agents of control. Everyday encounters with professionals routinely left them with a sense that they were not listened to. For example, they commonly wanted to talk through life experiences, including experiences that had prompted the onset of mental illness, but found these opportunities limited in statutory mental health services. On the other hand, we were told stories of men being expected to act independently once they had passed particular care thresholds. Regaining agency should be viewed as an incremental process that may involve men learning or relearning the skills to look after themselves.

From individualism to collaboration

We have proposed a model of mental health recovery for Black men in the UK that involves men establishing safe spaces to be themselves, forming authentic relationships and a satisfactory social identity, and enacting agency. This is a gradual and ongoing process – a journey – that does not occur in isolation. Black men in the UK commonly experience life journeys in which they are expected to deal with ongoing physical, emotional and social threats as rugged individuals, which in itself may contribute to their mental health difficulties. We argue that recovery requires this cycle to be broken and for Black men to be able to engage in more co-productive practices across all areas of their lives.

Black men largely view their relationships with mental health professionals as controlling and unhelpful to their recovery. While professionals working in health and social care services are clearly committed to providing a positive experience to service users, organisational structures and culture afford only restricted opportunities for developing positive and meaningful relationships with service users. It is evident that the depersonalised scripts that professionals are obliged to use close down conversations that might enable Black men to contribute as experts by experience to their own care. Although clinical governance aims to protect the safety and wellbeing of patients (Halligan & Donaldson, 2001), it has resulted in shaping practice through compliance with regulations and protocols. The focus is often on algorithmic and task-based approaches directed towards the management and/or avoidance of risk. Patients and service users are variously categorised as dangerous, vulnerable, resilient, dependent, independent, guilty and innocent (Fisher et al., 2018). As things stand, professional practice in the NHS remains largely based on a zero-sum understanding of power that perpetuates and entrenches the privileging of professional knowledge over other forms of knowing, particularly the expertise of experience acquired by members of marginalised groups (Fisher, 2012).

Rose and Kalathil (2019) argue that such practices referred to above sustain professional knowledge and do not support coproduction. Black men want to be able to address issues personal to them, and in particular related to their own African and Caribbean culture, during their experiences with clinicians. Creating a safe space where a service provider and service user can meet, for example, requires a commitment that extends beyond a task-based approach to professionalism. Lwembe and colleagues (2017) suggest that cultural competence is achievable through coproduction. These authors further suggest that coproduction has potential for addressing inequalities in mental health. Hatzidimitriadou and colleagues (2012) found that coproduction can yield positive outcomes for communities and mental health services, but that this can only be achieved when systemic barriers are brought down. Likewise, we suggest that agency is not an attribute developed by individuals in isolation; rather, it emerges through relationships that support a person's sense of self-worth. This type of engagement is difficult to achieve in a service provision context that is largely shaped by biomedical definitions of mental illness and one in which providers may have few opportunities or time to stray from expected scripts of care. In our study, good practice was invariably identified as negotiated in relationships of coproduction that acknowledged and drew on Black men's own experiences, insights and expertise by experience.

Conversely, as previously discussed, in our study, peer support and men's support groups were overwhelmingly experienced as 'safe' and nurturing. The positive experiences that the participants in such groups benefit from suggest that recovery and the re-negotiation of identities are parallel and entangled processes that are achievable in relationships of solidarity. By focusing in an open and fluid way on the relationships, rather than on 'fixing' people, such men's groups appear to promote a culture where the focus is on 'recovery together', rather than on a deficit, 'service-recipient' model that perpetuates othering and is often experienced when accessing mental health services. Informal groups provide opportunities for blurring roles that traditionally separate patients from healers. Instead, they provide the emotional and social space to encourage mutually supportive relationships and the pursuit of meaningful activities. Through these processes, rigid identities, often embedded in traditional understandings of masculinity, become more open to a more fluid understanding of self that appreciates that autonomy is found within relationships of interdependence.

Conclusion

Relationships across all areas of life are important for recovery: relationships with family and friends, informal carers, with providers and with society more generally. However, Black men in recovery continue to face stigma, which denies them empathy, respect and social recognition from others (Bourdieu, 1984). There is a need for further education around mental health, such that Black men in recovery – indeed, anyone in recovery – feels safe and secure to form authentic relationships based on co-operation, collaboration and trust, rather than battling with perceived or actual expectations to cope by themselves. Services and professionals must evidence a genuine will to build trust in Black men by listening to them in order to understand issues from their perspectives, as opposed to the perspectives of services. It is notable that some of the men in our study would not nominate providers who supported their recovery journey due to issues of trust and misrecognition. However, with African and Caribbean men, there is a specific need for services to validate life histories that have often been blighted by personal and racialised trauma, misrecognition and oppression. We propose that this can be achieved through coproduction.

References

Bologh, R.W. (1990). *Love or greatness. Max Weber and masculine thinking: a feminist enquiry.* Routledge.

Bourdieu, P. (1984). *Distinction: A social critique of the judgement of taste.* Routledge.

Bridges, T. & Pascoe, C.J. (2014). Hybrid masculinities: New directions in the sociology of men and masculinities. *Sociology Compass, 8,* 246–258.

Brownhill, S., Wilhelm, K., Barclay, L. & Schmied, V. (2005). 'Big Build': Hidden depression in men. *Australian and New Zealand Journal of Psychiatry, 39,* 921–931.

Bury, M. (2002). Sociological theory and chronic illness: Current perspectives and debates. *Österreichische Zeitschrift für Soziologie, 27*, 7–22.

Cabinet Office. (2017). *Race disparity audit: Summary findings from the ethnicity facts and figures website*. Cabinet Office.

Care Quality Commission. (2013). *Monitoring the Mental Health Act 2012/13*. Care Quality Commission.

Davies, S. (2014). *Annual report of the Chief Medical Officer 2013. Public mental health priorities: Investing in the evidence*. Department of Health.

Department of Health. (2005). *Delivering race equality in mental health care: An action plan for reform inside and outside services and the government's response to the independent inquiry into the death of David Bennett*. Department of Health.

Fisher, P. (2012). Ethics in qualitative research: 'Vulnerability', citizenship and human rights. *Ethics and Social Welfare, 6*, 2–17.

Fisher, P., Balfour, B. & Moss, S. (2018). Advocating co-productive engagement with marginalised people: A specific perspective on and by survivors of childhood sexual abuse. *The British Journal of Social Work, 48*, 2096–2113.

Halligan, A. & Donaldson, L. (2001). Implementing clinical governance: Turning vision into reality. *British Medical Journal, 322*, 1413–1417.

Hatzidimitriadou, E., Mantovani, N. & Keating, F. (2012). *Evaluation of co-production processes in a community-based mental health project in Wandsworth*. Kingston University and St George's, University of London.

Honneth, A. (2001). Recognition or redistribution? *Theory, Culture & Society, 18*, 43–55.

Kuh, D. & Hardy, R. (2002). *A life course approach to women's health: Does the past predict the present?* Oxford University Press.

Lwembe, S., Green, S.A., Chigwende, J., Ojwang, T. & Dennis, R. (2017). Co-production as an approach to developing stakeholder partnerships to reduce mental health inequalities: An evaluation of a pilot service. *Primary Health Care Research & Development, 18*, 14–23.

Robinson, M., Keating, F. & Robertson, S. (2011). Ethnicity, gender and mental health. *Diversity in Health & Care, 8*(2), 81–92.

Rose, D. & Kalathil, J. (2019). Power, privilege and knowledge: The untenable promise of co-production in mental 'health'. *Frontiers in Sociology, 4*, 57.

Sainsbury Centre for Mental Health. (2006). *The costs of race inequality*. Policy Paper 6. Sainsbury Centre for Mental Health.

Slay, J. & Stephens, L. (2013). *Co-production in mental health: A literature review*. New Economics Foundation.

Sullivan, M. (2016). *The patient as agent of health and health care: Autonomy in patient-centered care for chronic conditions*. Oxford University Press.

Chapter 3

Collaboration in secure care: A history of the past, the present and the future

Mark Chandley and AB

'If collaboration is the answer, what is the problem?'
(Frank Riley, Director of Scottish Recovery Network)

This chapter focuses on the profound challenges of keeping true to ideals of coproduction within the totalising confines of high-secure mental healthcare. We maintain a critical and sceptical tone throughout, not because we are opposed to coproduction but because our experience has left us – a member of staff with a long career in such environments and a service user detained within them[1] – somewhat bruised in our respective struggles to navigate the obstacles we highlight. On the rare occasions that coproduction can be approximated within the limitations of secure care institutions, it is to be celebrated as a chink of light in the unrelenting darkness. If such flickers of co-operation and empowerment can be coaxed into life and sustained in the face of the forces that would snuff them out, then coproduction could certainly make an important difference, even in these designedly hostile settings. That said, our purpose here is to provoke and challenge, to raise some hell (Cahn, 2008). As such, our arguments are unashamedly polemical.

Creating relationships of mutuality with our neighbours is a general social rule in most cultures. Co-existence with others appears to be a primordial social

---

1. Throughout the chapter we will refer to our jointly held views. At turns in our narrative, however, it makes most sense to single out the unique service user perspective provided by AB.

need; relationships are part of a successful life. We ask that people think about this in the context of the social relationships that are possible within a secure hospital. For Goffman (1968), 'stigma' refers to being 'discounted' or 'not included', resulting in a 'spoilt identity'. A detained person almost inevitably experiences stigma, as they are considered doubly deviant (Pilgrim, 2018). There may even be a triple jeopardy of stigma: for the crime (in the public imagination, the darkest and most hideous crime), for the mental disorder, and for the associated social situation (Chandley, 2005). To survive and recover from such mortification, detained individuals need to renegotiate a positive identity or achieve a sense of redemption for previous acts (Coffey, 2012; Ferrito et al., 2012).

But secure care is a community of paradoxes that rarely make sense. Despite incarceration being widely understood as therapeutically inappropriate, graded restrictions are routinely applied to patients in secure settings. The social situation of being locked away, both cerebrally and physically, can diminish basic abilities to navigate implicit social rules. It can have physical effects such as weight gain, turning people into unrecognisable pastiches of their former selves. This is sold as therapy – very expensive therapy indeed, exacerbated, as the sickest and most vulnerable are segregated further. This is not the healthcare many staff signed up for. In its extreme, segregation is objectionable, paradoxically increasing exponentially but becoming acceptable in psychiatric culture.

We begin by examining how patients in secure care navigate relationships and how this becomes enmeshed with institutional appraisal of risk. AB states:

> Good relationships with staff have been really important to me, but I have found boundaries are different to different people. What some may see as banter, others will take [as] offence. Or what might be appropriate humour to some people may not be to others. Sometimes the line might get crossed, but this could be in an innocent way.

An accurate clinical note might well record this observation as a concern and refer it on to the multidisciplinary team. Then it is potentially reified and medicalised as evidence of dis-ease; converted to dangerousness over time. This is not malice; the staff group is simply orientated to highlight risk. That may affect discharge – the prize of the majority of those detained with no 'EDR' (earliest date of release). The discharge goal may not be collaboratively decided, as processes typically play out in shorthand, without the knowledge of the detained person. According to Edward Shils (1996), such practices occur casually in corridor discussions, break facilities and informal meetings. So, there is the time served and the 'bullshit' (oft claimed by patients) transforming the passing of time into 'enduring time'. It is akin to 'belonging to the peasant classes, kinships and rural settings' or the precedence of past time over the present and future time (see Gurvitch, 1964, p.91). So, your history is your present and future. Secure patients indeed live with a review of their past becoming the future. As Sartre (1969, p.109) explains: 'The past is continually organised with the present [...] the past can be reborn to haunt us, in short to exist for us.'

The importance of the relationship at the nurse–patient interface is taken for granted by practitioners and patients. Yet both limit their expectations in an equally 'taken for granted' manner. Being taken for granted, though commonplace, is an objection and often, but not always, translates into poor practice. The whole dynamic is reasoned as protectionist, precautionary and safe. The assurance that we are professionally safe and at the cutting edge, however, does not consider the often-contradictory impacts for people. Yet AB's comments above are salutary. He wants to relate but must navigate the official truth. Chandley (2005) describes how the temporal suspension of relationships seems like a 'time warp' to patients; or, as noted by George (1998): 'I live in hope but reside in limbo.'

Boundary breakers

In secure services, all relationships must have boundaries. Collectively, staff are arguably by far the most frequent boundary breakers. This emphasises the relative normality of boundary breaches, and the limited consequent social disgrace. Yet, as we have noted, detained people value relationships and collaboration with individual staff members, not the wider depersonalised establishment. The clinical notes phenomenon mentioned above reflects a coercive spectrum permeating every aspect of practice for the person in secure care. Thus, a single clinical note has power beyond its documentary contribution. Völlm and Nedopil (2016, p.3) state that coercive measures are a 'sliding scale of pressure to accept treatment'. This treatment is invariably, perhaps exclusively, biomedical. We might ask, if there were wider alternatives on offer, would scope for cooperation increase (McKeown et al., 2016)? Clinical notes and hospital slang often orient to an 'NHS newspeak' (Chandley, 2005; Richman & Mercer, 2004); a new hyper-real, technical language (Mason & Chandley, 1992) increasingly becomes the *patois* of a corporatising NHS.

A veneer of politeness prevails. Rarely is anyone critical, at least to your face; it can be quite hideous behind your back. Battles between professionals require further skills. They are best acknowledged by Shils (1996, p.ix) in his skewering of organisations:

> Gentle reader be not perplexed. You have not entered a hall of mirrors; you are not lost in a cave of winds. You have encountered nothing more commonplace than bureaucracy. Mind, I said don't be perplexed; I did not say don't be depressed.

Risk and recovery

It is reasonable to risk assess. We do not think this is particularly contentious. Yet, amidst the rhetoric of balancing risk and recovery, positive risk assessment in secure care is often an anathema, as is 'least restrictive option' – a central principle of the Mental Health Act 1983 Code of Practice (Department of Health and Social Care, 2015). Practice is paralysed by administrative processes tied to the risk of assault and the potential for public humiliation or litigation if someone gets it wrong. Consequently, the overall secure population grows, even if high-secure facilities have shrunk; a policy hastened by public inquiries and acknowledged failures of management that include two such inquiries of note led by Sir Louis Blom-Cooper QC (1992) and Peter Fallon QC (Fallon et al., 1999; Tilt et al., 2000).

Risk assessment is not like weather forecasting, based on algorithms, models and previous data. Unlike the weather, if high risk is predicted and a patient does nothing wrong, it will be reasoned that this is because of the excellent risk management and it will be applauded. So, risk assessment is almost always precautionary because of a requirement to remain professionally safe. The risk of a false positive is continued detention. The risk of a false negative is reoffending, with all the reputational damage that brings. There is an inbuilt tendency to risk aversion.

Additionally, as we have seen, clinical notes can become restrictive and dominant. An 'official truth' over time can extend detention. AB writes:

> I was coming up for a tribunal and noticed I had been recorded as having four incidents of verbal aggression. It turns out I swore. Where I come from it was mild, but I must have insulted someone. My point is that nobody told me, I was oblivious… until it came to my freedom.

Sometimes a risk might present at low frequency yet be severe when it does occur. The consequences of getting risk management wrong can be catastrophic for the unsuspecting clinician. When a detained person is transferred from one unit to another of lesser security, the receiving unit does not typically trust a risk assessment completed elsewhere. This results in a tightening of restrictions, so those detained complain that they are not allowed a TV, leave, a phone or whatever small 'privilege', when they were before. Paradoxically, every unit worth its salt will claim to be working in partnership, will pay homage to coproduction and declare this on its noticeboards. Professional rhetoric or newspeak or bullshit? You decide. 'Do no harm' is the first canon of most ethicists, yet the unsuspecting detained person must navigate this predicament with the skill of a master. There is no redress. Silence may be the correct course. Not for too long, though, or you could be diagnosed as reclusive and isolating. Risk management processes are in need of risk assessment. It should be a coproduced enterprise, and perhaps then it might be more effective.

An Orwellian experience

Secure care in the UK has a distinctly Orwellian and dystopian character (Chandley, 2005). Promotion for staff relies on ritualistic compliance with the dominant truth, to be repeated like a paternoster. Senior managers believe everything is perfectly fine, that they are providing 'excellence', because they are officially rewarded. One tactic is to use the term 'culture' pejoratively in describing the workforce, specifically to undermine dissenting viewpoints. In Orwell's *Nineteen Eighty-Four* (1949), Newspeak is the language devised by the totalitarian government to replace 'Oldspeak'. It may not be hyperbole to suggest modern mental health organisations symbolise Orwell's totalitarian, oppressive state. Collaboration is often conflated with compliance, with biomedicine and corporate truth. Perversely, most patients are rarely engaged in collaboration as their opinion is an uncomfortable irritant to established corporate and psychiatric truths.

Tensions exist between those who explain the world through Newspeak and those relying on Oldspeak. This chapter might be heretical for Newspeakers. The problem is not just how they speak; rather, their language organises the world and their mind. Those who speak Newspeak believe it. With language, we create a world, not describe it (Garfinkel, 1967). Organisational leaders and their disciples thus happily and unthinkingly discursively reproduce the status quo.

Ward nurses are not able to renegotiate discursive and physical restrictions. They are hemmed in by rules, dominant truths and statutory bodies constraining all room for manoeuvre. In our experience, this has been the case for some considerable time (Mason & Chandley, 1992), and remains true today: a generation of lethargy, lack of change and organisational indolence. Honest negotiation should be the beginning of collaboration. We find ourselves constricted and controlled by mental health law and accompanying codes of practice that allow for the plague that is the isolation of seclusion, segregating patients from others and their rights. This legislation works against collaboration by legitimising coercion. This is not collaboration; it is a national disgrace.

Ever since the 1980s, we have heard people proudly proclaim that secure patients are part of a hospital community, yet they clearly reside in a total institution (Goffman, 1968). The patient group is affronted because they cannot be a citizen. They are not listened to. They are the subject of 24/7 surveillance, observed by staff and CCTV. They have little/no choice and have no family life. Some community!

When one of us asked a group of patients in high-secure care if they saw themselves as citizens, the responses made for sobering reading:

- I cannot vote.
- I cannot work.
- I still have duties beyond my sick role, I cannot provide for family.
- I cannot have any intimate relationships/sex.
- I cannot earn money.
- There is no way I can pay tax.
- Pension – this was talked about a lot as no one knew if you could pay into a private pension if incarcerated.
- I cannot have a meaningful marriage even if married.
- I do not have any liberty/freedom.
- I cannot drink/smoke.
- I cannot walk freely in the open air.
- I am locked up at 9pm, irrespective of my need.

Pilgrim (2018) claims that elements of recovery are not possible for interned people due to their involuntary status. He contrasts two ideas: the principle of coercive psychiatric practice versus coproduction and the idea of citizenship with this cohort of people:

> The citizenship of the service user will be respected: this simply does not happen under conditions of psychiatric detention. (p.271)

Severely restrictive practices

Perhaps secure services are those places most obviously resonant with the panoptical systems of control and surveillance highlighted by Foucault (2012). From the perspective of a detained person, the experience of being restricted might begin with segregation, being locked in a room for a significant period. The location of such detainment is irrelevant. Beirut? A Soviet gulag? The urge to be released is usually palpable and immediate.

It is hard to find much mutuality in power relationships enforcing internment against a person's will, with nearly 4,000 people detained at different levels of secure care. Despite avowed practitioner ideals of therapeutic relations and relational security, high-secure environments privilege physical security measures that bolster the symbolic separation of stigmatised inmates from the community at large: them from us. There may be some legitimacy of commitment with diminished responsibility for a serious offence, but this need not automatically necessitate blanket institutional rules such as night-time confinement or seclusion practices. Perhaps some of the initial decision-making around individual episodes of seclusion is sensible (minimising violence), and there may even be some consensual entry into seclusion, but this gets lost in institutional failures to end seclusion, and the segue into segregation.

Speaking but not heard

People detained are referred to as patients, reinforcing Parsons' (1975) 'sick role', medicalising, and reducing autonomy, telling detained persons what is best for them. That is not equal by any standard, not 'least restrictive practice' (Department of Health and Social Care, 2015). It is coercive, hidden in the rhetoric of the official truth. What Mason and colleagues (2008) perceived as foreclosure, as censorship, plays out. Again, it demonstrates institutional indolence, even as society has moved on. We succeed in cocooning people with paternalistic laws and codes. We continue to ignore social texts and evidence. Secure psychiatry is reduced to a biopsychological view of the world. This is not progress or enlightenment. This confident foreclosure is entirely ignorant of the survivor groups' experience whereby the principle of 'equal rights, equal voices' is championed. Secure detainment is officially reified into 'your community', institutional living as a 'choice'.

There were three people in two high secure special hospitals in long-term seclusion in 1996 (Mason et al., 1996). The exponential growth in segregation across services is problematic. It correlates to austerity, to underfunding. It indicates that these people are not considered equal to a similar physical healthcare group in intensive care. In the aftermath of the funding crisis that will follow Covid-19, there may be scant hope for the future. A fresh, critical look at what constitutes 'least restrictive practice' is required. Each deterioration into segregation points to a failure of law, code of practice, or statutory body to lead in a manner consistent with the principles mandated by the shorthand of the so-called Mandela Rules,[2] or the UN General Assembly (1984), or its Committee Against Torture (2018).

---

[2]. The United Nations Standard Minimum Rules for the Treatment of Prisoners. See www.un.org/en/un-chronicle/nelson-mandela-rules-protecting-rights-persons-deprived-liberty

Again, we argue for a future without undue restriction, a change of paradigm. We assert that the law is essentially unfit for the coming decades, that secure care is too costly and causes more harm than good. We have seen more employees become ill, physically harmed, drink alcohol to excess, take drugs, require the support of supervision and wellness courses, be sick, need re-education, require camera surveillance, become emotionally pained and relive traumas. Foucault might smile wryly and say, 'I told you so.' He would liken secure care to post-industrial gulags. The 'no EDR', or no way of estimating the end of detention, should be contracted in law, so the detention length is defined and transparent, linked to progress, with obligations on either side so an observable trajectory might be explicit from admission. This would support a system relying on detainment to one that is about responsibility and timely healthcare.

Who am I?

> I am a patient who is currently in a low-secure unit in the north-east of England. I have made my way through from high secure, down to medium and now to low. I am a father, son and brother and husband. I am in hospital because I was violent; I committed an act of violence whilst having a psychotic episode. The episode lasted for a couple of weeks. I have been in hospital now for over eight years. I am hoping to be back out and in the community shortly, in the next 18 months. I do think the length of stay in hospital is too long; however, I could have been released sooner, if it weren't for my own behaviour. Patients on the whole are frustrated with the length of stay they have to endure. (AB)

This account should have the reader ask: 'Is this detention reasonable?' A rebuttal would rightly consider both risk and danger to others – issues that should trump other practice considerations. Patients span from high secure (defined as 'a grave and immediate danger' in the Mental Health Act, 1983) to low secure (patients broadly defined 'as a significant risk' (Centre for Mental Health, 2011)). On closer examination, it appears that we may have added to the stresses of detention, forbidding a detained person to deal with family duties that continue to exist into detention, if not isolation. Would that cause a reasonable person stress? Partners and family life become a sideshow, collateral damage, while the Newspeak of the importance of relationships is exposed. Despite there being often no risk to family, sexual relationships are outlawed in many levels of detainment, leaving the detained person to build new relations when he leaves. This seems unjust, unfair and restrictive to us; introverted and antisocial.

Intimate relationships attract sanction

Despite the official mantra that relationships are key in secure care, these environments (with possibly rare exceptions) neglect existing relationships, such as with families (McKeown et al., 2019). Instead, these are regarded with suspicion, neglecting any sense of appreciation for traumatic disruptions in lives. Families and friends, including married people, are expected to maintain a family life and obligations but receive little support for this.

> Not so long ago, an old girlfriend of mine got in touch through my family. They gave her the hospital's phone number and told her where I was. She got in touch; I was really happy as we had always remained friends. We started to build a relationship over phone calls. During one particular phone call, she asked me if I needed anything bringing up – I told her I was 'okay'. She insisted she wanted to bring me something. She came to the hospital and handed a bag to reception. The next thing I know, I am called into a room with my doctor, my psychologist and a nurse. They explained that a woman has turned up at reception with a bag containing underwear and T-shirts. I said 'Yes, it is a friend of mine (well actually an old girlfriend).' I was put under real pressure; interrogated over a selfless act from a good friend. One said, 'Nobody just gives you something without getting something in return! Have you pressured her to give you these expensive gifts?' and 'She must expect something more from you.' This even dragged out into my weekly psychology sessions. The whole experience made me very reluctant to carry on whilst I was in hospital, so I phoned her and tried to explain. I was also a bit embarrassed about the whole thing, I told her about the way my care team reacted. It put me off having any relationship with her, which is really sad. I will get back in touch with her when I am released and who knows whether we will end up as partners or stay as just friends. (AB)

How can we speak of the importance of relationships and then outlaw an intimate relationship and, likewise, proclaim ourselves collaborative? The definition of a relationship is monopolised by the expert-by-profession and imposed on the detained person. Marriages, an essential protective bond in Western society, are discounted. They are, however, highly relevant to life beyond detainment. By whose standard can this be called collaborative? The binary question of inclusion or exclusion is interesting. Compliance is highly valued among staff as well as involuntarily detained people. To break with tradition is to be perceived as deviant.

Anyone deviant in secure care is, by Becker's (1963) definition, an 'outsider'. At the beginning of this chapter, we asked the reader to think: are you an 'insider' because you are compliant, or an outsider because you question, you think? Becker (1963, p.4) famously said: 'It is easily observable that different groups judge different things to be deviant.' Where, we ask, do you belong? On the one hand, we expect society to be sensitive, which is a good thing, part of how a civilised society is measured. Yet, a relationship is outlawed and frowned upon as dangerous. It must be kept secret or left to rot in the name of blanket restriction. Following Blom-Cooper (1992), an internal report recommended more liberal marital conditions (Taylor & Swan, 1999), but this was shelved, prioritising safety over relationships (Cohen, 2011). A contemporary review of relationships is urgently required in secure care in light of societal change.

Power and relationships

The NHS Constitution (Department of Health and Social Care, 2015) mandates a set of values congruent with continued employment in health services. Often, in practice, values and opinion are confused in the pursuit of compliance with the next audit result. Dissent is dealt with by a series of causal contingencies, all designed to foreclose that perspective. Mass compliance among colleagues stifles thought, imagination and creativity. This, we argue, is entirely restrictive and completely coercive. It leaves little space for deliberation around each other's opinion, so collaboration with the detained has no practical example. Few people officially acknowledge the collective compliance dynamics of 'silencing' and 'foreclosure'; 'keeping your mouth shut', whether you are patient or staff, represents a rational survival tactic in the face of organisational power. Such power is wielded by orchestrating both 'silence' and 'foreclosure' as coercive social control in an unconscious, insidious and secretive manner, often transacted at a collective level, regardless of the characteristics of individuals. Arguably, everyone experienced in secure services is aware of the controlling phenomenon of silence and foreclosure, colloquially known as 'keeping your head down' or 'keeping below the parapet'. As Kesey (2005, p.32) emphasises, 'There's a whine of fear over the silence.'

Nevertheless, as Marx (1859/1904, p.11) would contend, 'It is not the consciousness of men that determines their existence, but, on the contrary their social existence determines their consciousness.' It follows that collective reasoning changes with the audience (social group), and this is an observable phenomenon. Hence, compliance only occurs in the social group it is acceptable in. Never elsewhere! A person could, in these settings, variously hear the oft-used phrase, 'But he would say that', aimed at a difficult patient or staff – usually a casual comment, negative, loaded with personal important messages about value and worth and deployed to undermine that person's point of view. It points to a weakness, be that illness, intelligence (or lack of), past or present failures, indecencies or infidelities. At once, this is existentially undermining of the person, by pointing at their spoilt identity; the stigma attached and now cemented.

Freedom of speech

> I learned very early on in my stay in hospital to keep my mouth shut. My speaking out about things, I later found out that it had been reported that I am argumentative and inflexible. I myself would disagree with that, as would anybody who really knows me, so I now walk a very fine line. You get punished but are told punishment doesn't happen. But it clearly does, because if you are not walking that fine line, things will get held back. For example, leave getting postponed – this will make for a longer stay, whether you are well or not. (AB)

Silva and Shepherd (2019) comment on detained people's inability to object to the restrictive practice of night-time confinement. They state: 'Curiously, most patients do not complain, either informally or otherwise, and some report feeling safer.' It is, again, taken for granted foreclosure. However, in rebuttal, AB states that he learned to 'keep his mouth shut. It is a skill'. In fact, voicing concerns attracts informal sanctions. It is not worth it for most and often leads to a variety of protest behaviours, which is odd, given the official duty of care of secure facilities in England.

It is regrettable that one of us cannot reveal his identity – the very soul of self. His personal focus is on discharge and he is obliged for the sake of his future liberty to remain anonymous. (He fears sanctions.) In fact, he wants to remain in the shadows; in other words, to keep his mouth shut. Surreptitious restrictive practice is part of the spectrum of poor practice that costs a great deal, both fiscally and socially. We ask, is this restrictive? Is it the wish of a civilised society? Is it dutiful? We mean, 'to keep our mouths shut'?

A small fortune is spent on this internment, creating a net surplus of mental disorder rather than a reduction. We are not curing illness, but producing it – a curious, expensive, postmodernist twist. Are we motivated to change, or will it take another significant period of time to change? Will we wait, like before, for external scrutiny and suffer the indignity of being told that we are not good enough, or will we make our own demands for fundamental reform?

Conclusion

Notable commentators on recovery, Boardman and Roberts (2014, p.18) assert: 'Changing traditional ways of doing things in any organisation is difficult.' We concur. Until the Mental Health Act or guidance changes, the law on incarceration as a method of delivering healthcare is non-negotiable. Paradoxically, we are signatories to the Mandela Rules. Professionals are caught in what Heller (1961) calls 'a Catch 22'. It is our duty to follow the law; the issue is, which one? Until we relax security and reduce coercion, we are recovery restricted. Staff optimism alone cannot carry a concept or organisation. We require clarity around these subjects, a civilised dialogue grounded in humane healthcare, where possible coproduced with the patients.

We provide recommendations in hope rather than expectation. The early 19th-century progressive reforms of at the Salpêtrière asylum in Paris and The Retreat in York were followed soon after by regression and continued indolence. We expect secure care will follow the same path – a cyclical trajectory that will be the subject of continued critique. We can reflect that our secure hospitals may one day be preserved as museums to detainment, to non-compliance to the Mandela Rules and the United Nations rules on torture (UNCAT, 2018). They will be theme-parked, with tour leaders showcasing seclusion rooms with tales of inhumane treatment and questions of the workforce about segregation and how the mentally disordered could have gravitated to this in a period of collaboration. What did the staff do? We will have followed rules ('I was doing my duty'). We are reminded of a quote by Oppenheimer (1955, p.115):

> It is not only honourable to doubt; it is mandatory to do that when there appears to be evidence in support of that doubt.

We should review the secure contract and legislation to help the vulnerable. We should be thinking about further appropriate reform and review of the Mental Health Act. If coproduction represents a new paradigm, then we must legislate for this. Done properly, coproduction will save money. The current thin veneer of collaboration is riddled with serious rights issues. The breaking of the Mandela Rules, to which the UK is a signatory, is breath-taking. We should begin with respect and depart from an unhelpful 'without limit of time' to a trauma-informed contract with obligations on both sides. This should bind patients and staff to various elements. The accompanying code of practice should facilitate freedoms and solutions and support healthcare professionals to authentically enact coproduction, not offer guidance antagonistic to international ideals. Fringe and 'radical' groups should have a say and sociology should be at the heart of conversations around future provision.

This requires investment, money and quality staff trained in secure provision. Seemingly open-ended segregation should be outlawed as a disgrace, outdated and inhumane, not masqueraded as healthcare, at least not in our name. Or, at minimum, we should work out a more precise set of circumstances where it may be justified and always seek to minimise duration. We should decide if we want to be collaborative and not allow the colonisation of corporates to delude the world with rhetoric. We must allow practitioners to ply their profession, but allow for a greater plurality of ideas, including the sociological. We should look internationally at what others are doing to liberate the mentally disordered and the emancipatory demands made by psychiatrised peoples.

We are aware that we are but little cogs in a big machine. We speak 'a truth', but not 'The Truth'. At least this chapter is a record of our views. There is definitely more to come with regard to the truth. So, returning to the question on collaboration: 'If collaboration is the answer, what is the problem?'

References

Becker, H. (1963). *Outsiders: studies in the sociology of deviance*. The Free Press.

Blom-Cooper, L. (1992). *Report of the Committee of Inquiry into Complaints about Ashworth Hospital*. The Stationery Office.

Boardman, J. & Roberts, G. (2014). *IMROC Briefing 9: Risk, safety and recovery*. Centre for Mental Health/Mental Health Network.

Cahn, E. (2008). Foreword: A commentary from the United States. In L. Stephens, J. Ryan-Collins & D. Boyle. *Co-production: A manifesto for growing the core economy*. New Economics Foundation.

Centre for Mental Health. (2011). *Pathways to unlocking secure mental health care*. National Mental Development Unit.

Chandley, M. (2005). *Temporal experiences in a special hospital: A multi-method, qualitative study of socio-temporality at Ashworth Hospital*. [PhD thesis.] Manchester Metropolitan University.

Coffey, M. (2012). Negotiating identity transition when leaving forensic hospitals. *Health*, *16*(5), 489–506.

Cohen, S. (2011). *Folk devils and moral panics: The creation of mods and rockers*. Routledge.

Department of Health and Social Care. (2015). *Mental Health Act 1983: Code of practice*. The Stationery Office.

Fallon P., Bluglass, R., Edwards, B. & Daniels, G. (1999). *Report of the Committtee of Inquiry into the Personality Disorder Unit, Ashworth Special Hospital (Vol. 1)*. The Stationery Office.

Ferrito, M., Vetere, A., Adshead, G. & Moore, E. (2012). Life after homicide: Accounts of recovery and redemption of offender patients in a high secure hospital. *Journal of Forensic Psychiatry & Psychology, 23*, 322–344.

Foucault, M. (2012). *The birth of the clinic*. Routledge.

Garfinkel, H. (1967). *Studies in ethnomethodology*. Polity Press.

George, S. (1998). More than a pound of flesh: A patient's perspective. In T. Mason & D. Mercer (Eds.), *Critical perspectives in forensic care: Inside out* (pp.102–107). MacMillan Press.

Goffman, E. (1968). *Stigma: Notes on the management of spoiled identity*. Penguin.

Gurvitch, G. (1964). *The spectrum of social time*. D. Reidel Publishing Company.

Heller, J. (1961). *Catch 22*. Black Swan.

Kesey, K. (2005). *One flew over the cuckoo's nest*. Penguin.

Marx, K. (1904). *A contribution to the critique of the political economy* (N.I. Stone, Trans.). Charles H. Kerr & Company. (Original work published 1859.)

Mason, T. & Chandley, M. (1992). Nursing models in a special hospital: Cybernetics, hyperreality and beyond. *Journal of Advanced Nursing, 17*, 1350–1354.

Mason, T., Henighen, M., Chandley, M. & Johnson, D. (1996). Decompression from long-term seclusion. *Psychiatric Care, 3*(6), 217–225.

Mason, T., Mercer, D. & Richman, J. (2008). Professional convergence in forensic practice. *Australian and New Zealand Journal of Mental Health, 10*(2), 105–115.

McKeown, M., Jones, F., Foy, P., Wright, K., Paxton, T. & Blackmon, M. (2016). Looking back, looking forward: Recovery journeys in a high secure hospital. *International Journal of Mental Health Nursing, 25*(3), 234–242.

McKeown, M., Jones, F., Stewart, S. & Foster, S. (2019). Family support and involvement in secure mental health services. In N. Evans (Ed.), *Family work in mental health: A skills approach* (pp.83–102). M&K.

Oppenheimer, J.R. (1955). *The open mind*. Simon & Schuster.

Orwell, G. (1949). *Nineteen eighty-four*. Secker and Walburg.

Parsons, T. (1975). The sick role and the role of the physician reconsidered. *Millbank Memorial Fund Quarterly, 53*(3), 257–278.

Pilgrim, D. (2018). Co-production and involuntary settings. *Mental Health Review Journal, 23*(4), 269–299.

Richman, J. & Mercer, D. (2004). 'Modern language' or 'spin'? Nursing, 'newspeak' and organizational culture: New health scriptures. *Journal of Nursing Management, 12*(5), 290–298.

Sartre, J.-P. (1969). *Being and nothingness: An essay on phenomenological ontology*. Routledge. (Original work published 1943.)

Shils, E. (1996). *The torment of secrecy: The background and consequences of American security policies*. Elephant Paperbacks.

Silva, E. & Shepherd, A. (2019). Editorial: Tick, tock, lock: Night time confinement in high security – history, practice, ethics and practicalities. *BJPsych Bulletin, 43*(1), 1–3.

Taylor, P. & Swan, T. (Eds.). (1999). *Couples in care and custody*. Butterworth & Heinman.

Tilt, R., Perry, B., Martin, C., McGuire N. & Preston, M. (2000). *Report of the review of security at the high security hospitals*. Department of Health.

UN Committee Against Torture (UNCAT). (2018). *General comment No. 4 (2017) on the implementation of article 3 of the Convention in the context of article 22*. UNCAT. www.refworld.org/docid/5a903dc84.html

UN General Assembly. (1984). *Convention against torture and other cruel, inhuman or degrading treatment or punishment*. United Nations. www.refworld.org/docid/3ae6b3a94.html

Völlm, B. & Nedopil, N. (Eds.). (2016). *The use of coercive measures in forensic psychiatric care: Legal, and practical challenges*. Springer AG.

Chapter 4

From depression to delight and nearly everything in between: A non-academic perspective

Elaine Harrison

This chapter is about how I got to where I am, coproducing and being coproduced!

In my younger days, I was very confident, believing that I could independently do anything and that I was good at it. Now, my confidence has diminished; I wonder, has what have I done with my life been worthwhile? Who would want to read this 'twaddle'? But we are all worthy and all have something to contribute. I am sure that, if I strike a chord with just one person, then it is worthwhile. Unless you 'feel the fear and do it anyway' (Jeffers, 1998), you will never achieve anything worthwhile.

So, here is my story, in 15 episodes and a postscript.

No. 1

It began in 1964, when two people coproduced me. It had worked successfully in 1961 when they produced my brother. My life began on a January evening; it was a normal and happy childhood. I was very conscientious and worked hard at school. However, I went to pieces at exam time and unfortunately my results showed the great angst I must have had. I dreamed of being a teacher but, lacking the necessary qualifications, the dream was shattered. I was bewildered, fed up and did not know what to do. I remember, at that time, I was ready to procrastinate for the rest of my life.

No. 2

It was then that my first big coproduction started. My dad took it upon himself to get a prospectus from Southport College. Together we hatched a plan and I enrolled on a secretarial course. This was my first experience of doing something for 'each other'. Dad did all the research; I turned up on the course and gave it my all. It proved to be a great course, where I met lots of people. At the end of the course, we were assigned two weeks' work experience. Had my Dad and I not coproduced this, then maybe I would still be procrastinating, who knows? My work experience was at the Liverpool School of Tropical Medicine. I was very fortunate to be offered a full-time job with them, and my journey into the big wide world began.

No. 3

I am stepping into the world of relationships – after all, is not this really what coproduction is all about: being there for each other, offering support and encouragement, a shoulder to cry on, a 'pick up' if you stumble? Someone to bounce ideas off, to share? This is my interpretation of coproduction, anyway. I find relationships such a roller coaster of emotions: good and bad. One minute you can be as 'high as a kite', floating on loveliness, and then as down as a dog, depressed because they have not phoned when they said they would. I think this is when we literally can change the passage of time: when we are with someone we love, time can pass by so quickly, hours seem like seconds, but when you are waiting to see a loved one, minutes can seem like hours. John was everything I wanted and more; he was the yang to my yin. But there was an issue.

No. 4

My first true love, John, was an exceptionally good mechanic and was soon headhunted down south. I was so much in love and so loved being a couple. His boss soon wanted to keep him content, and I was offered a job with the same company. There I was, living 'down south', cohabiting, coproducing wonderful happy memories. Or were they? It was not long before John was not feeling 100% happy or even content and decided to move back to Liverpool. Very much the downside of coproduction: bewilderment, frustration, heartache.

No. 5

I was single! I call these the wilderness years: no partner, no family nearby; no one to coproduce with; just existing, not really enjoying life. Okay, I had a good, well-paid job, but with the financial rewards came the responsibility and demands to produce results. It became very stressful and no one was there for me: no one to share, no one to care. I felt I was a withering flower. The stresses and strains became unbearable and I was very unhappy indeed. It was then that I fell into that deep dark hole I could not get myself out of – some may say a rut, but this was deep depression. I was alone, very alone, no hope, no way out. What would be my next coproduction?

No. 6

A friend turned up late at night. She was trying to attract my attention through the window, trying not to alarm me. Though a little startled, I was surprised to see her. She had had an argument with her husband and had walked out in frustration and, in her words, wanted to teach him 'a bit of a lesson'. We sat and chatted. She told me about a course that she had just finished that she had enjoyed immensely; she had gained huge benefits from it. She told me it was expensive but worth every penny, and it might be something I would like too. I phoned for more details and decided to start the course. When I looked at the paperwork, it was a 'Diploma in Hypnotherapy, Psychotherapy and Counselling' from the School of Analytical and Cognitive Hypnotherapy (SACH), based in Essex. I was a little apprehensive about the word 'hypnotherapy'. Did I really want to be involved in that? During my very dark days, I would turn to reading; books became my friends and I could enter a new world. I admit many of them were 'self-help' books. Some were invaluable. It was a treat to go to a bookshop and let the book choose me. It became addictive. But addiction is a negative word, right? No, this was a healthy addiction; they were getting me better and it felt great. One of my favourite authors is Betty Shine. Her titles appealed to my imagination. I read *Mind Magic* (1992) and was hooked. I would read each day; it was my tonic.

No. 7

The first morning of the course, I felt very apprehensive. I knew I could still back out. I had not paid upfront and I would not be letting anyone down at this stage, apart from perhaps myself. I picked up Shine's latest book, *Mind Waves* (1993). I read page 42 and turned the page. It was a new chapter entitled 'Hypnotherapy'. I just knew that I had to do the course. I picked up my coat, bag and keys and headed to the venue, feeling very apprehensive and nervous. Everyone was in the same situation. The tutors ushered us to our chairs, set in a horseshoe, and introduced themselves. I can still remember to this day, after nearly 18 years, a tutor saying, 'I'm nervous and excited, and it is exactly the same feeling.' He was right. You could tell the tutors were very good friends and this was coproduction at its very best. The course ran for 12 months and I had to create 100 case studies. I enjoyed it so much that I went on to do the advanced course. I have made life-long friends and learnt life-long skills. The course was very intense at times. You felt you were really delving into people's intimate issues; you felt privileged that they trusted you with their feelings. It was draining and you would go home exhausted. During this course, I had my 'light-bulb' moment. We touched on laughter and how good it was for you. I decided to create my own laughter workshop, but I knew I could not do this on my own. I did not have the confidence. I needed to coproduce, but with whom?

No. 8

Pam was a lovely lady, a fellow student on the course, very experienced. She was more mature. She had been a midwife, had worked for the Marriage Guidance Council and The Priory, a national private-sector mental health provider. She regularly had clients and was well established. She was very encouraging and supportive and instilled confidence in me. She thought my idea was wonderful, and that is why we went ahead. I would never have done this on my own. We met regularly to figure out what we thought would work. She showed me how to have structure and professionalism. It was during one of our coproduction meetings that she said that her friend had given her (comedian) Ken Dodd's telephone number and maybe we should ask him for some advice. Without further ado, she was phoning the number and we could hear his answerphone come on. 'Hello, Mr Dodd, we are planning a laughter workshop and wondered if you could offer any advice for us.' I was giggling at the surrealism of it all. I think it must have only been 10 minutes and her phone rang. It was the man himself. How 'tickled' was an understatement. Younger readers, you will have to google that!

No. 9

So Laughter Factor was born. A friend of mine suggested writing to the local newspaper in Billericay, Essex, to advertise the date. I did not want to pay for an advert so I sent an email saying that readers may be interested in a new innovative group that would benefit people, improving their wellbeing and making friends. The plan worked. We were on page three of the local newspaper. How exciting; our 15 minutes of fame had started. The newspaper promised that they would follow up the next week to see how it all went.

The date was set, the invitations despatched, the nerves had kicked in, or was it excitement? The day before, Pam and I were just doing last-minute preparation when the phone went. 'Hello, can I speak to Elaine Harrison? This is Jenny from ITV television. My boss came in this morning and said: "I just want something fun," and so I googled 'fun' and your laughter workshop came up.' I was perplexed at first but realised the newspaper had put it online.

She continued: 'I'd like to send the cameras down and film everything, would that be okay?' I was aghast, speechless. I had a good face for radio, but television was a completely different story. I was not ready for that, so I told her it was a pilot and perhaps next time. That is what thinking on your feet does for you, in a two-minute reaction time, sometimes you must make a life-changing decision. Although I had been in the Girl Guides as a teenager where the motto was 'Be prepared', I was not prepared for that.

No. 10

The day arrived. The balloons had been bought, the bunting put up. The day was beautiful and went very well. The concept was brilliant. The hall was filled with laughter, a wonderful magical sound that personally I think is heaven sent. The day was A-star, a huge success and full of memories for life. The newspaper kept their side of the bargain. A full-colour photograph appeared in the paper the next week. I felt like a celebrity. A lot of co-operation – coproduction – had been put into this event and we proved it worked. But what next?

No. 11

A rest? I was returning to procrastination. I had few friends and my family lived a long way away. I was lonely; I was at a crossroads. One way would lead me to depression, the other to a brighter future. I chose the latter. I became creative. When you are alone with your thoughts, it is amazing how ideas and projects come to mind. I had seen a beautiful leather bag in the charity shop – so unusual, very 1950s, but a very weird colour, lilac. It was too nice to throw away and, at only £1, I had to have it. The shape was beautiful, but it was just that colour!! It needed decorating, but with what?

No. 12

Saturday night and only *The X Factor* for company. Was this what my life had become? A bottle of wine and a packet of liquorice allsorts were summoned. I then decided that sweets were very colourful and just what my bag needed. I forgot all about *The X Factor* and started cutting up the sweets. They looked great, but a little something extra was needed. Yes – dolly mixtures would do the trick. I thought the result was fantastic. My 40th birthday was fast approaching, and it was my dream to have dinner at The Ivy, the world-renowned restaurant in London. I would take my totally unique and unusual bag with me. I got lots of compliments. I was sure this was how I was going to make my millions. Aware that this was unique, I feared it might get 'copied' and I would not get recognised as the creator. There was no *Dragons' Den* on TV then.

No. 13

I was watching the TV one morning when a competition advertised for 'crafters'. I listened as if the presenter was talking directly to me. 'This is it,' I thought, 'This is my moment.' I never normally like having my photo taken but I just knew my bags would be popular. I could not go on my own. I needed a companion, to give me confidence and put me at my ease. Who? Yes, Pam, the lady who had helped me with Laughter Factor. I phoned her and asked if she would go with me to the studios. 'Yes,' came her reply, and off we went. There were lots of like-minded people there, who'd brought cards and pictures, knitting, dolls' houses even, but nothing was as bright and unusual as my bags. I was quietly confident the first prize was mine.

I entered the room where the judges were sitting, two males and one female. I have this, I thought. The first gentleman was very kind. He said, 'It is a yes from me.' The second was a lady. Girl Power, I thought to myself. She is bound to say 'yes'. I could not quite believe my ears when she said, 'No, it is not for me.' Time stood still. Was I hearing her right? Had I become overconfident? The third guy, a young TV presenter for kids' art, perked me up and said, 'Yes, I think it is fab!' I was through to the next round. The end of the day came, and they announced who had won. I stood nervously, practising my 'Yes, I have got it' face and 'Oh no, I am disappointed' face. It was the latter, and I need not have practised. I was very disappointed. So what now?

No. 14

I had made lots of goods for the show and I did not want to bin them. After all, I had spent quite a bit of time and money on them. A friend of a friend had a stall at Greenwich Market, a local street market in south London. I asked myself, 'I wonder if that is where I should take my wares?' I asked him what he thought. He said it was a brilliant idea. The stall was £30 and £5 to park the car. Even if I did not sell a thing, I told myself, it was a day out. I followed this guy in his van and felt I was not alone. (Is this more evidence of coproducing at its best?) It was December 2005, a bright, cold day. I was all set up by 7.30am. Around 8.10am, a man came along with a younger person, perhaps his daughter. He announced that he thought my stall was wonderful and he had not seen anything quite like it; he must buy a picture. This was my first sale and I told him so. I asked if he wanted me to 'sign' the back. I felt sure that I would be famous one day and the Number One picture would be worth a fortune. We laughed. I think mine was more a nervous laugh as he handed me a Scottish £20 note. I was unsure if this was even legal tender. I had to give him one of my British £5 notes; I thought 'I could be out of pocket here.' I decided I did not want to offend him; he had been so complimentary.

No. 15

Christmas came and went. Dark and dreary January came. I heard the postie walk up the path. Plop. I had post. I opened the letter. Eek, it was from the credit card company. I had not paid my December bill and had a penalty. 'Yuck,' I thought, 'How miserable.' Just then the phone rang. 'Hello, I doubt you remember me. I bought something from you when you had your stall at Greenwich Market.' I replied, 'Of course, I do. I remember signing your picture as you were my first customer.'

'Well, I live in Scotland and there is a shop up here that wants to stock your items, is that something you think you could do?' Without hesitation, I instantly said, 'Yes, not a problem. What is the name of the shop?' 'Cloud Nine,' came his response, and yes that was exactly how I was feeling. Whoop, whoop.

We arranged to meet in a mutually safe area, definitely somewhere public, for my own peace of mind. I took a choice of items so he could take his pick. He bought well over £200 worth. I was absolutely delighted – over the moon, in fact. He asked what other arrangements I had for rest of the day and, without sounding too much like 'Billy-no-mates', I said no definite plans. He then asked if I would like to eat. Just then his mum phoned, and I could hear her saying she would make dinner and he asked me, would I like to go to his parents' house? I had to think on my feet. This was against my feelings of 'stay public'. I thought, 'This man could be a mass murderer or anything.' I do not know if he could tell what I was thinking but he suddenly said: 'No, let's go to Canary Wharf.' I thought, 'Phew, a much better idea. I could "remain public".'

We had a wonderful time. I could tell quite early on that I could trust this man. He was very comical and had me laughing all the time. I had those wonderful belly laughs that hurt your side sometimes. I realised that I had not laughed in such a long time and it felt so good. He was very generous. This man had the top two qualities I find very attractive in a man. Only, I did not find him physically attractive. He had longish, greyish, curlyish hair and, to be honest, I felt like something was living in it! Anyway, this was not a problem because I did not see him as a potential date, more a business partner!

He was originally from London. He frequently visited his family and had business in the City. He visited 'down south' quite a lot and was phoning me regularly. We became great friends. When he next came to London, I met up with him, but this time it was different; he had had his hair cut! Now, if you have ever seen the British TV programme *EastEnders*, this would be a 'dff, dff, dff' moment!

As I fast approach my allocated word limit, there is something I must tell you. A very special occasion happened where 'all my Christmases and birthdays came at once'. On 22 December 2006, I became a mother and had my beautiful daughter, Isla. Her father was my very first customer on 11 December 2005 and is officially known as my 'dream-maker'. Coproduction had come full circle.

Postscript

I used to have a very professional job, advising top executives in London, but unfortunately the strains and stresses eventually took their toll. Once I became a mother, the dream of all dreams, I almost became housebound and much engrossed in *Peppa Pig* (other children's TV programmes are available, lol), children's stories and Lego. I had almost forgotten what it was like to be 'adult'.

I first became formally involved in coproduction in 2015, when Julian Raffay presented a course at a recovery college here in Liverpool. I was accompanying my cousin, offering support both physically (as he does not drive) and emotionally. Not long after the course, Julian invited me to attend a Lived Experience Advisory Panel (LEAP) meeting. I did initially wonder why I was there and what it was all about. Julian assured me that I was a valued member and my thoughts and comments mattered, and that made me feel good.

The LEAP meetings gave me a chance to get suited and booted and feel 'professional' again, if only for a few hours. I gave my time freely, but the one proviso was that this time must be within school hours; I must be able to drop my daughter at school and collect her at three. I surprised myself that I had the confidence to make suggestions and delighted that they always accommodated me. I enjoyed these meetings. I was given the opportunity to speak openly and never felt humiliated or embarrassed. It did absolute wonders for my confidence and welcomed me back to some sort of professional world again.

I can remember when Julian announced that he had been approached to write a book and wanted to involve us all. I instantly found this a very exciting opportunity and knew that I was among experts who knew what they were doing, and it would be fun and informative to feed off their expertise and experience. Julian is an amazing guy and is definitely 'the glue' in this whole process of bringing us all together. I know that if this book you are holding right now was titled 'Glue', you would find it hard to put it down! Get it? Great to end on a laugh!

References

Jeffers, S. (1998). *Feel the fear… and beyond: Dynamic techniques for doing it anyway*. Vermilion.
Shine, B. (1992). *Mind magic*. Corgi.
Shine, B. (1993). *Mind waves*. Corgi.

Navigating coproduction: Conclusion

Julian Raffay and Pamela Fisher

The authors in this section have argued that coproduction is not a quick fix nor an elegant solution. Unlike Einstein's $E=mc^2$, coproduction does not explain what was previously found bewildering. On the contrary, it is an invitation to resist applying formulae, and perhaps even definitions, to human distress. Coproduction invites a paradigm shift from Newtonian mechanics (where A implies B implies C…) to one where we confront the complexities of our shared humanity. If we embrace coproduction, we will surely find ourselves 'treading on holy ground'. No one is sole expert. Even more bewildering, we are all experts with invaluable perspectives.

Coproduction settles differently

For we editors, the most noteworthy aspect of these chapters is the need to recognise that coproduction settles very differently for different people. Some find themselves in positions where they can get involved without risk of harm. Others fear withdrawal of their treatment or actual malice. Several professionals who started out with us felt unable to continue, for fear of recrimination. Some service users and carers had to withdraw because of deteriorating health or increasing responsibilities. We were particularly aware of 'intersectional discrimination', where those most vulnerable to discrimination are most at risk (Bartley, 2017).

A problem of scale

One stark possibility is that titanic institutions (in every sense of the word) are intrinsically hostile to coproduction (Moore, 2017). We are disturbed by market-driven NHS trust takeovers that leave staff distracted by endless reorganisations and ever more distant command-and-control structures. Inevitably, these shiny projects promise heaven on earth, but we have found things very different on the ground. Staniszewska and colleagues (2012) show what happens when stakeholders become marginalised:

> The outcomes of involvement seemed to be predominantly defined by the organisations involved rather than service users, so we know relatively little about the outcomes that service users wanted to achieve. Such difficulties challenge the notion of true partnership, as certain groups dominate the ways in which methods, context or process are decided. (p.138)

Coproduced partnership may call for more 'pleasant processes' (Halliburton, 2003), potentially better served by small local clinics than by the anonymous bureaucracies of technical medicine. In 1978, the economist Schumacher argued that we need to build on a human scale where people feel they matter. We may wonder how anyone who does not feel cared for themselves might be able to sustain the demanding task of caring for others. No one can survive in an 'emotional desert', neither service user, nor carer, nor staff (Raffay, 2020, p.102).

Pioneering has the two-steps-forward, one-step-back quality echoing the take-up of all-electric cars. Redefining or recalibrating success may help us avoid losing heart and move progressively forward, albeit more slowly than we might have first hoped.

Although coproduction may at times appear simply too much effort, our experience has convinced us that the alternatives are no easier. Pretending there is life in the 'broken and demoralised system' (Schizophrenia Commission, 2012, p.4) is exhausting for all concerned. We may feel as if we are lighting up these dark places with nothing more than a few candles. However, lighted by their flickering, faltering flames, we see just enough to reach forward, step by step. Most importantly, we have shown the terrain that advocates of coproduction are navigating. A key question might be whether coproduction should concentrate on outputs (coproduction in its strictest form), outcomes (co-evaluation), or processes (involvement).

In the next section, we move from isolated accounts of stakeholder experience towards a more systematic exploration of barriers and facilitators. We avoid oversimplifying or suggesting sure-fire methods, as these very approaches may be the problem we are trying to leave behind.

References

Bartley, M. (2017). *Health inequality: An introduction to concepts, theories and methods.* Polity Press.

Halliburton, M. (2003). The importance of a pleasant process of treatment: Lessons on healing from South India. *Culture, Medicine and Psychiatry, 27*, 161–186.

Moore, G. (2017). *Virtue at work: Ethics for individuals, managers and organizations.* Oxford University Press.

Raffay, J. (2020). *The relationship between mental health services and faith communities: A co-produced grounded theory study.* [Doctoral thesis.] University of Durham.

Schizophrenia Commission. (2012). *The abandoned illness: A report from the Schizophrenia Commission.* Schizophrenia Commission.

Schumacher, E.F. (1978). *Small is beautiful: A study of economics as if people mattered.* Abacus.

Staniszewska, S., Mockford, C., Gibson, A., Herron-Marx, S. & Putz, R. (2012). Moving forward: Understanding the negative experiences and impacts of patient and public involvement in health service planning, development and evaluation. In M. Barnes & P. Cotterell (Eds.), *Critical perspectives on user involvement* (pp.129–141). Policy Press.

Section 2

Barriers and facilitators to coproduction

Barriers and facilitators to coproduction: Introduction

Catherine Mills and Mick McKeown

This section introduces some of the barriers and facilitators to coproduction. If innovatory practices that are more inclusive, participatory and democratic are to survive and thrive within modern mental health services, then the supporters of coproduction need to be acutely alert to factors that might sustain or impede progress. Such progress, after all, is in everybody's interests, but perhaps not everybody will be a supporter, let alone an evangelist for change. The seductions of professional power and status can strongly militate against sharing them. Thus, the status quo might prevail, despite the appeal of more rewarding work as a democratic professional.

Furthermore, even staff inclined to embrace the democratic promise of coproduction might mistrust the sincerity of any organisational affinity for the notion. This may be especially the case if previous attempts at democratisation of care relationships have failed to deliver authentic and meaningful change. Many such staff may also wryly note their relative disempowerment within employment relations typified by hierarchical command structures, close disciplinary surveillance, denuded pay and job security, and high levels of sickness absence and attrition of the workforce. In such circumstances, innovation and change of any sort can flounder amidst the vicissitudes of insufficient, or even safe, staffing levels. Idealised forms of work can appear unrealisable when faced with an everyday reality of 'catching your tail and firefighting' because of insufficiency of resources (McKeown et al., 2019).

Potential allies in service user and survivor movements may remain powerfully sceptical that meaningful democratisation can occur or is even on offer. Progressively inclined staff may indeed share in this cynicism. Other colleagues may simply be exhausted by any proposed changes to working practices that appear to land as prescriptions from on high into a morass of perpetual 'change', where nothing much actually changes at all. All concerned may feel worn down by previously ineffectual struggles to avoid the co-option and dilution of previous great hopes for radical change, such as 'user involvement', 'shared decision-making' and 'recovery'.

Obstacles to change are many. Lack of staff or organisational support for innovation can manifest in various ways, ranging from indifference, through assorted forms of resistance, to out-and-out sabotage. Service users disempowered by sundry coercions and restrictions can find it difficult to be persuaded into a more co-operative standpoint within essentially mistrusted services. Perhaps the most obvious barrier facing a mission to democratise mental healthcare is the fact that, despite a degree of softening over recent decades, these services remain organised around a quite singular and, for some, oppressive, biomedical approach. This is enmeshed with societal demands for public safety such that mental health professionals, far from any democratic ideal, are actually bound up in a risk-averse system concerned primarily with the control and containment of disruptive or dangerous 'mad' people. In this sense, it is the public and government who are best considered the 'users' of mental health services, rather than the individuals we refer to as 'service users' (Rogers & Pilgrim, 2014). Recognising this demands that we consider the potential to democratically transform mental healthcare through a wider societal lens, as much as focusing on change within services themselves.

From a societal perspective, we must acknowledge the prevailing unhelpful impact of neoliberalism and the recent politics of austerity. A series of governments committed to retracting the state, privatising welfare institutions and public utilities, and promoting a cult of individualism at the expense of more collective, mutual relationships has contributed to undermining faith in public service. An unholy trinity of government, the mass media and unfettered multinational corporations, with perhaps government as the junior partner, are complicit in a corollary that is undermining of faith in democracy itself (Crouch, 2011). It seems that, under austere neoliberalism, those citizens who have most to lose or gain in our democracies are the least likely to exercise their democratic rights and cast a vote in elections. Not unrelatedly, with an increasingly shaky conceptual foundation (Glas, 2019) and public scandal over failures of care, including startling examples of neglect and abuse, faith in psychiatry is also diminished (Roberts & Ion, 2014).

Citizens and welfare service users seeking a democratic voice amidst such powerful countervailing social forces might seem to be terminally disempowered and unrepresented. Yet, out of the ashes of these crises of legitimacy, sparks of resistance and claims for participation will always emerge (Habermas, 1981). Thus, mental health system-survivor and service-user social movements make demands that both result from the legitimacy shortcomings of psychiatry and represent cogent means for transformation of the crisis. These are essentially demands that speak truth to psychiatric power, seeking a more even distribution of this power: a call for democratisation that recognises the hard fact that 'power concedes nothing without demand, it never has and it never will' (Douglass, 1857, pp.21–22). At one and the same time, such social movements could be an alternative to coproduction, working independently of the state and services, or a powerful ally in achieving coproduction ideals across services. The latter prospect also might involve political and practice-based alliances with critically minded staff and their representative organisations, such as trade unions, opening up the possibilities for a new, democratic professional identity (Dzur, 2019).

Despite the various impediments to coproduction, the idea for more cooperative and democratic means of organising and delivering public services has been around for some time now (Ostrom & Ostrom, 1977), and has resulted in some notable successes in unlikely places (Dzur, 2019). The chapters included in this section all, in various ways, show how extant barriers have been, or can be, surmounted to offer coproduced services or enact relevant meaningful change across different settings. In doing so, they illustrate the supportive factors necessary for sustaining coproduction and highlight opportunities for making a start.

Chapter 5, written by Rhiannon Corcoran, Maureen Thomas and Julia Zielke, looks at meaningful spaces for people who experience a low sense of worth. Such spaces might include neighbourhood hubs and other community settings, and integral to this are the processes involved in creating these facilities and spaces. This chapter explores our human capacity for pro-social relationships and how the use of coproduction methods relates to outcomes and success. Three strands are addressed: relational wellbeing, relational spaces and relational design. The authors look at how coproduction struggles to thrive within a hierarchical system and requires the democratisation of space. Ultimately, the process of democratised design may prove more important than the outcome.

Coproduction and care planning within mental health services is explored in the next chapter, by Catherine Mills, with key examples drawn from one NHS trust. Chapter 6 takes a look at the historical aspects of care planning over the years, moving on to current practices and the barriers experienced in today's settings. Three very different types of service are studied: a female acute ward, an assessment ward for people with dementia and a male high-secure ward. Coproduction is balanced against a need to incorporate factors such as risk and safety (of self and others). It also looks at the role of carers in care planning and coproduction within a triangle of care.

Next, Lucy Webb and Amanda Clayson offer a chapter dealing with coproduction within addiction services, addressing some of the specific challenges of working with this client group, who may be socially excluded and alienated. Chapter 7 offers an example of coproduction and participatory research in a healthcare setting – The Recovery Voice in Action project. This introduces a data-collection tool called VoiceBox. The clients in recovery became the VoiceBox 'crew' and outline here their experiences and reflections on the process. The chapter concludes by comparing coproduction in fields such as environmental sciences with that in healthcare and what learning can be achieved from this.

Chapter 8 turns to coproduction in a forensic learning disability service and is co-authored and coproduced by a research practitioner, Michaela Thomson, and two people who use and access an NHS forensic service, writing under the pseudonyms Mike Hargreaves and Shaun Peterson. This chapter challenges current ideologies and thinking around working alongside people with a learning disability. It offers an account of how to successfully coproduce, giving practical examples (e.g. the use of Easy Read materials), with the service user co-authors actively contributing to the process, and this writing partnership emerging out of a long relationship in practice. The chapter concludes with top tips for the involvement of people with a learning disability in genuine coproduction that could be extended across services.

The section concludes with a really practical demonstration of how to break down barriers to coproduction, based on the experience of the author, Kate Pieroudis, of working at the Social Care Institute for Excellence (SCIE) and other disability organisations. Chapter 9 explores the practical and philosophical barriers to coproduction. It describes distinctions between simple involvement, through consultation, to true coproduction. It suggests solutions to extant barriers, based on events and discussions between people who use services and professionals. There is a thorough exploration of issues such as power-sharing, legislation and policy, attitudes, organisational culture, money and resources and accessibility.

This section encompasses a broad range of ideas, concepts, exploration of specific exemplar services and discussion points about coproduction and how it can be achieved in the real world. Actual practice is emphasised in real-world settings, which will hopefully inspire the reader to take on the challenges and barriers to achieving coproduction and share in its successes in practice.

References

Crouch, C. (2011). *The strange non-death of neo-liberalism.* Polity Press.

Douglass, F. (1857). *Two speeches by Frederick Douglass; one on West India Emancipation [...] and the other on the Dred Scott Decision.* C.P. Dewey, American Office. www.libraryweb.org/~digitized/books/Two_Speeches_by_Frederick_Douglass.pdf

Dzur, A.W. (2019). *Democracy inside: Participatory innovation in unlikely places.* Oxford University Press.

Glas, G. (2019). Psychiatry as normative practice. *Philosophy, Psychiatry, & Psychology 26*(1), 33–48.

Habermas, J. (1981). New social movements. *Telos, 49*, 33–37.

McKeown, M., Thomson, G., Scholes, A., Jones, F., Baker, J., Downe, S., Price, O., Greenwood, P., Whittington, R. & Duxbury, J. (2019) 'Catching your tail and firefighting': The impact of staffing levels on restraint minimisation efforts. *Journal of Psychiatric and Mental Health Nursing, 26*(5-6), 131–141.

Ostrom, V. & Ostrom, E. (1977). Public goods and public choices. In E.S. Savas (Ed.), *Alternatives for delivering public services: Toward improved performance* (pp.7–49). Westview Press.

Roberts, M. & Ion, R. (2014). A critical consideration of systemic moral catastrophe in modern health care systems: A big idea from an Arendtian perspective. *Nurse Education Today, 34*(5), 673–675.

Rogers, A. & Pilgrim, D. (2014). *A sociology of mental health and illness.* OUP/McGraw-Hill.

Chapter 5

Relational spaces for mental health and wellbeing

Rhiannon Corcoran, Maureen Thomas and Julia Zielke

Even though the concept of coproduction originated in community-level initiatives, the translation of these ideas into a mental health service context has often neglected mental health-promoting possibilities and the wider community. This chapter offers such a focus, with an emphasis on key relational aspects of place and space within our communities. Understanding the role of places and spaces in the mental health and wellbeing of individuals and communities is a growing area of cross-disciplinary research. This chapter aims to examine relational concepts of wellbeing, space and design with a view to establishing how we can create places that address poor wellbeing, afford coproduction and facilitate meaningful activity in the context of mental distress. Examples from different perspectives and sectors are offered to illustrate established or innovative practices.

Wellbeing and community involvement

Following a scoping review (Bagnall et al., 2017) examining what works to improve social relations in our communities, the Community Wellbeing Evidence Programme of the What Works Centre for Wellbeing[1] produced a systematic review of published evidence addressing the question, 'Can

---

1. The What Works Centre for Wellbeing is part of the UK Government's What Works Network, which aims to improve service and provision in an evidence-informed way. https://whatworkswellbeing.org

we improve social relations and community wellbeing through community infrastructure?' (Bagnall et al., 2021). From more than 21,000 titles and abstracts of publications published in English between 1997 and 2017, 51 met the criteria for inclusion in the review. These comprised, among other things, studies that examined the wellbeing effects of community hubs, local neighbourhood interventions, urban regeneration and place-making. The review showed that the processes used to arrive at the output were equally, if not more, influential than the actual end product itself. This finding was brought into sharp focus because no evidence was found of wellbeing benefits to the community when interventions were delivered in an entirely top-down fashion, while wellbeing benefits were documented when there was meaningful community involvement in the planning and delivery of the intervention.

The team followed this review with another exploring the wellbeing impacts of shared decision-making in communities (Pennington et al., 2018), expecting to find uplift in community wellbeing when people were involved meaningfully in decision-making processes. While evidence did support this expectation, what was more telling was the finding that tokenistic involvement of communities in decision-making about their places actually led to negative wellbeing impacts, with people feeling ignored, side-lined and frustrated. In other words, when trust was compromised in the process, people felt bad. The evidence pointed to the critical factor at the heart of this failure of trust as being the quality of the established relationships between the powerful, in-charge change-makers and the relatively unempowered receivers of change, who felt the effects of having things done to them and done to the places they loved – their homes.

The idea that outcomes need to be collectively derived and value driven (e.g. to result in wellbeing benefits), and to meaningfully involve users of the service in the process, is fairly mainstream now. However, that does not mean that implementing this effectively is commonplace. Different contexts and environments put different and complex strains on establishing a practice of coproduction, and many might say that the context of mental health service delivery is among the most challenging. As other chapters deal with these particular challenges, we will not dwell on them here. Instead, we focus on how relational spaces can afford relational wellbeing and meaningful coproduction.

For all our good intentions to put wellbeing at the fore as an outcome of change, if we are to progress in a way that can more predictably produce wellbeing benefits for communities, then we need to better understand its core ingredient: relationships. In other words, in order to understand which kinds of wellbeing interventions produce which kinds of outcomes, we need to understand *how* different individuals, social groups, institutions and the living environment relate to one another. Rather than looking at single interactions and outcomes, we need to start looking at these relations as a process that unfolds in different spaces at the same time. Understanding how mental health relates to coproduction, beyond tokenism, inevitably includes a need to critically appraise the relational notions of a) wellbeing, b) space and c) design. This chapter attempts this by picking out the relational aspects of all three of these thorny concepts, using examples and evidence to illustrate its discussion.

Relational wellbeing

At its simplest, wellbeing can be understood as a state of feeling good and functioning well. The notion of relational wellbeing developed as a critique to what has been termed the 'component approach to wellbeing' (Atkinson, 2013), which simplified the complexities of human life as lists of measurable, static, fixed, separated components that can be added up to determine someone's wellbeing. This approach may consider the role of social connections but only as 'context', rather than as a mutually constitutive part of the human experience (Campbell & Cornish, 2014). Nikolas Rose (2019) has described this approach as the 'molecularisation of mental health', linking a quasi-mechanical understanding of the human brain and mental health to advances in neurochemical research and the rise of big pharma.

To illustrate, Michael Marmot starts off his book *The Health Gap* (2015) with a captivating example of his experiences on a psychiatric ward in Australia in the 1960s. A depressed woman enters the clinic. She says: 'Oh doctor… my husband is drinking again and beating me, my son is back in prison, my teenage daughter is pregnant, and I cry most days, have no energy, difficulty sleeping. I feel life is not worth living' (p.1). Marmot recounts that, at the time, all the doctor was able to say or know was how to diagnose 'a red pill-deficiency' (p.2), resulting in her changing from her 'blue pills'. But for Marmot 'it seemed startlingly obvious that her depression was related to her life circumstances' (p.2) and that red or blue pills could only address the symptoms but not the causes of the woman's depression.

Over the past four decades, a number of influential publications like Marmot's Whitehall studies on the social determinants of health (Marmot et al., 1991), *The Black Report,* showing how ill health is unequally distributed (Townsend & Davidson, 1982), and Brown and Harris's studies on the social origins of depression (Brown & Harris, 2012) have set the tenor for critical studies in public mental health. More recently, Wilkinson and Pickett (2010) further demonstrate how poor wellbeing strongly correlates with socio-economic inequalities, political uncertainty, austerity politics, neoliberal work regimes and our immediate physical and social surroundings. In short, how well we feel is not (only) a matter of our own inner dispositions but is also indicative of external structures that determine our chances of a 'good' life.

A more far-reaching form of this argument asserts that wellbeing can only be properly understood as a relational construct that embraces the evolved social nature of our species; that we need to be with and give and receive from others in order to realise a sustained sense of feeling good and function well reliably, day to day. A more relational approach between individuals and collectives, their formal and informal networks, issues of trust and reciprocity and questions around power and control (Prilleltensky & Prilleltensky, 2007) may also affect other people's and non-human animals' wellbeing in unforeseeable ways. Taking this model, then, makes it meaningless to separate wellbeing from its context of communities, environments and socio-politics. Those who adhere to the concept of relational wellbeing emphasise that wellbeing emerges from multiple interactions across time and space, and is more than the sum of its parts (Andrews & Duff, 2019; Atkinson, 2013; Atkinson et al., 2019; Smith & Reid, 2018; White, 2010, 2017).

A relational understanding of wellbeing puts communities into focus, asking what it means to feel good and function well *together*. Atkinson and colleagues (2019) argue that community wellbeing is not simply the sum of individual wellbeing but may feel more like the *function* of individual wellbeing. However, it can be understood better still as an emergent environment coming out of a sense of cohesion or togetherness, across time and space, sometimes referred to as 'we-ness' (Corcoran, 2017). Our innate prosocial tendencies are the basis of our 'success' as a co-operative species. We have an unparalleled, though not unique, ability to form cohesive groups. Developed and sustained from empathy, groups devise their own distinct cultures and ways of being.

These deep-rooted human processes are at work wherever we come together to make changes to our environments in order for people to flourish. Nevertheless, it is this relational wellbeing that is eroded by neoliberal and global capital policies that rely on the individual being footloose and free to serve the economic machine and derive their meaning and purpose from that service via the pursuit of personal wealth and growth (White, 2017). Under a capitalist paradigm, our own sense of personal worth can be linearly traced back and quantified through the hours we work, the wages we are paid and the goods we can buy to show this worth. Marxists speak here of species alienation – the idea that a sense of self is coupled to oppressive labour structures instead of derived from a sense of companionship, community and sense of empowerment (Harvey, 2017). In this sense, individual wellbeing in Western capitalist economies can be understood as being founded on *economic doing*, and relational wellbeing on *human being*.

Relational spaces: involvement and creative exploration

Creating environments in which we can flourish also brings into focus the importance of physical spaces in fostering wellbeing. As with wellbeing, we need to understand space as more than just a map-like, static, fixed background to our existence (Massey, 2005). However, there seems to be some reticence when it comes to defining relational space. Helpfully, Thrift (2003) offers the following definition:

> This is a relational view of space in which, rather than space being viewed as a container within which the world proceeds, space is seen as a co-product of those proceedings. (p.96)

In other words, spaces are not an inanimate background on which life 'happens' and objects 'are'; rather, relational space conditions and is conditioned by the way we live and interact with one another. In a relational understanding of space, what is *experienced* in space and what space *is* become largely synonymous. In this vein, space is social and imaginative – a canvas on which life is painted as an unfolding social practice. By widening the spaces for interaction, we allow a wider range of experiences to come together, because by bringing a diverse set of experiences together, we widen the space for new and different social and public possibilities. We see examples of relational space in makerspaces[2] and collaborative practices, which Wulf (1989, 1993) envisaged as 'centers without walls'. The broader literature refers to such relational spaces as supporting a wide range of human activity and meeting a broad range of human need, from minority-culture deliberative democracy (Gorman-Murray & Nash, 2014) to children's out-of-school activities (Thiel, 2018), for example.

With Thrift's definition in mind, we can play with the example of opening up, widening and sharing (public) spaces in the built environment. Such widened spaces can attract more diverse and democratic participation of marginalised and vulnerable voices and are pivotal in conceiving of relational spaces in the context of community wellbeing and mental health services. The following introduces two examples of doing so.

Example 1: Shared spaces in traffic

In traditional traffic spaces, there exists a clear hierarchy of users, with people in motorcars on the top and pedestrians (and cyclists) at the bottom. The introduction of shared space dissolves that hierarchy by reverting everyone

---

2. A makerspace is a collaborative work space within a school, library or other public/private setting for making, learning, exploring and sharing. See www.makerspaces.com

back to the level of citizen within a relational space – no longer a driver, cyclist or walker in a road space. Conceived originally by Monderman, a Dutch highway engineer, as a way of increasing public safety, shared space works (in a way that appears paradoxical to many) by removing the demarcations and signage used to guide the actions and behaviours of those using the space. Monderman has argued that what these markings and symbols in fact do is to isolate individual users within the space so that they come to be concerned only with their own movement and not that of other users. Indeed, as their own actions are prescribed by infrastructure that tells them how they must behave, each individual mover loses ownership over their own movements. Removing the signage and markings works to make individuals more aware of their own and others' movements in the space and, in doing so, increases the individual's sense of responsibility for actions and agency. In Monderman's words:

> We're losing our capacity for socially responsible behaviour [...] The greater the number of prescriptions, the more people's sense of personal responsibility dwindles. (Cited in Toth, 2009)

The reader might care to look at the video *Poynton Regenerated*[3] to see how this shared space has broken down the disconnection between drivers and other street users by reinstating civility in the car-dominated urban environment, as evidenced in the video by eye contact and hand gestures.

Essentially, shared space is democratised space that reinstates our natural human means of communicating with one another within what has become a hostile and dangerous, systemised environment. The environment, formerly managed as an apersonal traffic movement system, has been re-empathised. A re-empathising of the often brutal spaces meant to support mental health has been called for over many years by the survivor movement, with activity within the survivor collective itself being shown to support further recovery (Chassot & Mendes, 2015).

Example 2: Places of creative exploration and arts practices

Relational spaces emerge from within or across areas of activity when deliberative discussions are opened up that include all those who can claim a stake or an interest in the service or the area of activity.

Mo's House was one such idea that emerged in a series of three open meetings around improving mental health undertaken deliberatively within a large National Institute for Health Research (NIHR) programme grant (CLAHRC-

---

3. www.youtube.com/watch?v=-vzDDMzq7d0&feature=youtu.be

NWC). Mo's House, conceived by co-author Maureen Thomas, is a physically situated and relationally informed 'home' to support families and individuals, young and old, who are currently experiencing distress. Founded on principles of mutuality and trust, Mo's House merges the scales at which relational spaces and wellbeing operate. It is conceived simultaneously as homely, embedded within its community, and having the aim to serve unmet social and healthcare needs in the region. The aim of offering comfort, care, company and community across generations reinforces the operation of the house as family. As such, the benefits for looked-after children moving from traditional 'care' settings and for isolated elders may be particularly profound. With trust built up via communal activities drawn from the assets of Mo's House residents themselves, the hierarchical barriers to relational wellbeing are removed.

Like the concept of Mo's House, James' Place[4] arose from a national relational wellbeing need for support for young men in times of mental health crisis. James' Place is a community initiative sited close to a cluster of university campuses – areas with high support needs among young men who feel suicidal. It is a Georgian townhouse designed to provide a safe haven during crisis, and both its physical spaces and its social and therapeutic functioning are co-designed with those who find respite there.

Arts-based practices seem naturally to embrace relational ways of being and becoming well across different scales, from the individual to the communal, and so can provide effective practice that allows relational spaces to emerge and thrive. Zielke (2019) has used Story Houses, a method that combines poem writing and the crafting of a metaphorical home, as a way to collectively dwell on the complex layered experiences of mental health service users. She found that opening up spaces to relate to oneself and the environment through material and literary evocations and metaphors can help mental health service users take a nuanced look at themselves in their specific social, emotional and political context. Arts-based methods like the Story House give creative autonomy to the creator and also enable them to safely distance themselves from the immediacy of a painful moment.

'Madlove: A Designer Asylum', led by British artist and mental health activist James Leadbitter, is a more widely known example where arts-based practices were the catalyst to the emergent relational space that shifted thinking about how an asylum space can best serve those who either need or choose to use it. This reconnects with one of the original, more positive, meanings of asylum, as sanctuary – itself a concept redolent with issues of place and space (The Vacuum Cleaner, 2020).

---

4. www.nspa.org.uk/members/james-place

> It ain't no bad thing to need a safe place to go mad. The problem is that a lot of psychiatric hospitals are more punishment than love […] they need some Madlove.
>
> Is it possible to go mad in a positive way? How would you create a safe place in which to do so? If you designed your own asylum, what would it be like? […]
>
> Together we are attempting to create a unique space where mutual care blossoms, stigma and discrimination are actively challenged, divisions understood, and madness can be experienced in a less painful way. This temporary structure will be a reflexive and responsive space for exploring and redesigning madness.[5]

This work, along with the now well-established philosophy that underpins the Soteria network,[6] are examples of how mental health services can be re-empathised by engaging users of services in a levelled-up decision-making and governance model.

Another successful practice of wellbeing emerging within relational space is what happens during shared reading. The Reader Organisation[7] takes serious literature to a wide range of communities, from looked-after children to mental health services and prisons. We-ness emerges as groups of people connect with each other, using the book or the poem as their cornerstone. Such emotionally live group experiences, where the point and the purpose are to re-familiarise with self, learn about others and master literature, scaffolded by trusted light-touch facilitation within a safe and democratic space, are hard to find in everyday life.

Relational design: Democratising spaces for wellbeing

Relational notions of space may help us foster and build spaces for mutual understanding, care and appreciation of individual people's stories and histories. However, the question remains: how do we actually create such relational spaces? And how do we make sure that the relational spaces we create do not perpetuate the ways that power and influence are distributed in our traditional public processes? This is especially pertinent given that spaces of wellbeing are not neutral or evenly distributed. Indeed, under an austere and neoliberal climate, vulnerabilities are unevenly distributed across space in a way that often

---

5. www.thevacuumcleaner.co.uk/madlove-a-designer-asylum
6. www.soterianetwork.org.uk
7. www.thereader.org.uk

reinforces particular hierarchical power structures within society. A person can readily design and enact change at the scale of their home. A community group, assuming a degree of tenacity and effective cooperation, can enact change at the level of neighbourhood. However, only those operating at a larger scale of place (cities, regions, nations) have the readily resourced power to bring about structural change. Relational spaces also differ according to the level at which they operate, because different in-groups will be invited in, while out-groups will be kept at arm's length or ignored. Coproduction will therefore struggle to thrive within a hierarchical system and so the active democratisation of space must occur to enable it.

We argue here that the processes of relational design provide a way towards democratising relational spaces for wellbeing.

Blauvelt (2012) defines relational design as being:

> ... preoccupied not just with design's form or meaning, but with its effects; not with isolated objects, but rather with situations embedded in everyday life. (p.43)

Relational design therefore is founded on a social logic, involving end users in a process of 'designerly thinking'. So, relational design emphasises the process of design over the final product in a way that is consistent with the findings of the systematic review conducted on how place and space infrastructure can support community wellbeing, referred to at the beginning of this chapter. Blauvelt goes on to argue that:

> While most 20th century design is autonomous, independent, isolated, and closed, relational design is synonymous with interdependence, connectedness, and openness. (2012, p.48)

Example 3: Coproduction

Conceived in the first instance by Nobel Prize-winning economist Elinor Ostrom, in response to addressing discord on the streets of Chicago during the 1970s, coproduction as a means of delivering change has been taken up across diverse sectors. In the context of public services, the New Economics Foundation (NEF) defines it thus:

> Co-production means delivering public services in an equal and reciprocal relationship between professional, people using the services, their family and their neighbours. (NEF, 2010)

Because we are a social species, we naturally coproduce, but we tend to do so with our own in-groups. Coproduction is much more challenging when we have to co-operate with those who we perceive as 'out-group' members, or as being *not like us*. Thus, our prosocial tendencies, evolved as sources of adaptive fitness in our natural 'units', can be sources of tension and disharmony when systems make demands on us to coproduce across units. Those units, or perceived in-groups and, by extension, out-groups, might be the service providers and the service users. Therefore, working from within current systems, it is by levelling up power and democratising space that we can overcome the inevitable challenges of coproduction across groups.

Building on Blauvelt's proposition, as well as other examples of relational space, we propose that the design of relational spaces to assist further coproduction and to create relational wellbeing in the context of mental health services needs to foreground a process rather than a product in a way that:

- understands the human need to be social and to form trusting relationships
- is non-hierarchical, to level up power imbalances
- is context specific, so that standardised solutions cannot simply be imposed
- is agile, flexible, dynamic and evolving, because relational design does not stop with an output and relational wellbeing is an emergent property of interactions across time and space
- is open to and respectful and tolerant of difference, understanding the need for it before consensus, because there are many ways of being human
- is open to experiences and to the wide views coming from diversity
- is always encouraging, to establish trust
- is willing to take risks, because sometimes ideas will fail and we can always learn from failure.

Example 4: How a relational design process produces a relational space

Accepting the premise that, as a social species, we prefer face-to-face interactions to those that may take place in virtual relational spaces, it is worth spending time thinking about how relational spaces to support coproduction and mental health and wellbeing might happen. To illustrate, operating in the Liverpool City region, Mersey Care NHS Foundation Trust has driven award-winning innovation in the form of their Life Rooms. These, beginning with the co-design of space, have embraced service user need for a safe community space where they can engage in activities that are themselves coproduced, as well as meet up for the intrinsic purpose of being with others. As both a community provision and a commissioned mental health and wellbeing service, the three Life Room sites owned by the trust begin with a mentality of homeliness, using biophilic design principles when possible, while traversing the scales of space from home to community to region. With a focus on prevention, non-medical treatment and stigma reduction, the Life Rooms can only function through coproduction and so they have been designed using relational principles.

In achieving future relational wellbeing, relational design needs to be guided by the loftiest and most gestalt of the design principles – that of harmony: the sense that there is a belongingness of one thing to another. Although applied most commonly in visual design, harmony encapsulates the togetherness of the relational approach.

The co-design of place and space supports relational wellbeing by being an inherently optimistic process because, in making changes to spaces and places, the intention is always to create positive outcomes (Corcoran et al., 2018). The co-design of space using the relational approach supports not only the wellbeing of those involved in the process but also that of the wider and future beneficiaries of those relational places and spaces, because, at its best, it produces harmonious outcomes.

Example 5: Re-thinking the welfare state through design thinking

When, after the Second World War, the UK conceived its welfare state (including our NHS), our institutions could not possibly have foreseen the challenges services are facing today: families locked out of society, increasing chronic conditions, youth loneliness and an ongoing housing crisis that widens the raft of socio-economic inequalities across our communities. In today's society, the welfare state has become an affair of managing and controlling the silos of our social and healthcare systems that are supposed to address the needs of the most vulnerable in our society. But this system is no longer working, as our needs become so complex and entrenched and people are suffocated in a managerial miasma of already underfunded services.

According to Cottam (2015), we need to redesign the welfare state, starting with a capabilities approach. 'What is it that you want to achieve in your life and how can we help you get there?' is the sort of question at the heart of a capability-building approach. This starts by removing any top-down managerial intervention from services and giving patients and citizens room to breathe and think about what they actually want (rather than what they are told to want). Giving autonomy to the most vulnerable helps them regain control of their life and appreciates that there are no one-size-fits-all relational wellbeing solutions.

Conclusion

By examining the inter-relationships between wellbeing, space and design that emphasise the relational, a route towards the realisation of places that support mental health and wellbeing using democratic processes comes into focus. With plenty of pioneering work to support this aspiration, all it needs is for a concerted and shared will and trust to be built across currently divergent 'stakeholders' so that social and physical harmony results.

References

Andrews, G. J. & Duff, C. (2019). Matter beginning to matter: On posthumanist understandings of the vital emergence of health. *Social Science & Medicine, 226*, 123-134.

Atkinson, S (2013). Beyond components of wellbeing: The effects of relational and situated assemblage. *Topoi, 32*(2), 137-144.

Atkinson, S., Bagnall, A.-M., Corcoran, R., South, J. & Curtis, S. (2019). Being well together: Individual subjective and community wellbeing. *Journal of Happiness Studies, 21*, 1903-1921

Bagnall, A.-M., South, J., Di Martino, S., Mitchell, B., Pilkington, G. & Newton, R. (2017). *Scoping review: Social relations.* The What Works Centre for Wellbeing. https://whatworkswellbeing.org/wp-content/uploads/2020/01/social-relations-scoping-review-final-jun17-corrected.pdf

Bagnall, A.-M., South, J., Di Martino, S., Southby, K., Pilkington, G., Mitchell, B., Pennington, A. & Corcoran, R. (2021). *Spaces, places, people and wellbeing: Community hubs and green space.* https://whatworkswellbeing.org/product/places-spaces-people-and-wellbeing/

Blauvelt, A. (2012). The rise of the relational: Five themes in relational design. *The Journal of Design Strategies, 5*(1), 42-48.

Brown, G.W. & Harris, T. (Eds.). (2012). *Social origins of depression: A study of psychiatric disorder in women* (Vol. 2). Routledge.

Campbell, C. & Cornish, F. (2014). Reimagining community health psychology: Maps, journeys and new terrains. *Journal of Health Psychology, 19*(1), 3-15.

Chassot, C. S. & Mendes, F. (2015). The experience of mental distress and recovery among people involved with the service user/survivor movement. *Health, 19*(4), 372-388. https://doi.org/10.1177/1363459314554313

Corcoran, R. (2017). *Academic perspective: When communities of place become communities of interest: the magic catalyst of community wellbeing?* What Works Centre for Wellbeing. https://whatworkswellbeing.org/blog/academic-perspective-when-communities-of-place-become-communities-of-interest-the-magic-catalyst-of-community-wellbeing/

Corcoran, R., Walsh, E. & Marshall, G. (2018). The benefits of cooperative place-making: A thematic analysis of co-design workshops. *CoDesign, 14*(4), 314-328.

Cottam, H. (2015). *Relational welfare.* [Online.] www.hilarycottam.com/practice/relational-welfare/

Gorman-Murray, A. & Nash, C.J. (2014). Mobile places, relational spaces: Conceptualizing change in Sydney's LGBTQ neighborhoods. *Environment and Planning D: Society and Space, 32*, 622–641.

Harvey, D. (2017). *Marx, capital, and the madness of economic reason.* Oxford University Press.

Marmot, M. (2015). *The health gap: Challenges of an unequal world.* Bloomsbury.

Marmot, M.G. , Stansfeld, S., Catel, P., North, F., Head, J., White, I., Brunner, E., Feeney, A., Marmot, M.G. & Davey Smith, G. (1991) Health inequalities among British civil servants: The Whitehall II study. *The Lancet, 37*, 1387–1393.

Massey, D. (2005). *For space.* Sage.

New Economics Foundation (NEF). (2010). *Right here, right now: Taking co- production into the mainstream.* New Economics Foundation.

Pennington, A., Watkins, M., Bagnall, A.-M., South, J. & Corcoran, R. (2018). *A systematic review of the evidence on joint decision-making on community wellbeing.* The What Works Centre for Wellbeing. https://whatworkswellbeing.org/product/joint-decision-making-full-report/

Prilleltensky, I. & Prilleltensky, O. (2007). Webs of well-being: The interdependence of personal, relational, organizational and communal well-being. In J. Haworth, & G. Hart (Eds.), *Well-being: Individual, community and social perspectives* (pp.57–74). Palgrave MacMillan.

Rose, N. (2019). *Our psychiatric future.* John Wiley & Sons.

Smith, T.S. & Reid, L. (2018). Which 'being' in wellbeing? Ontology, wellness and the geographies of happiness. *Progress in Human Geography, 42*(6), 807–829.

The Vacuum Cleaner. (2020). 5 Years of Madlove. *Asylum: The radical mental health magazine, 27*(1), 4–6.

Thiel, J.J. (2018). 'A cool place where we make stuff': Co-creating relational spaces of muchness. In C.M. Schulte & C.M. Thompson (Eds.), *Communities of practice: Art, play and aesthetics in early childhood* (pp.22–37). Springer.

Thrift, N. (2003). Space: The fundamental stuff of human geography. In S.L. Holloway, S. Rice & G. Valentine (Eds.), *Key concepts in geography* (pp.95–108). Sage.

Toth, G. (2009). *Where the sidewalk doesn't end: What shared space has to share.* Project for Public Spaces. www.pps.org/article/shared-space

Townsend, P. & Davidson, N. (Eds.). (1982). *Inequalities in health: The Black report* (Vol. 1). Penguin.

White, S.C. (2010). Analysing wellbeing: A framework for development practice. *Development in Practice, 20*(2), 158–172.

White, S.C. (2017). Relational wellbeing: Re-centring the politics of happiness, policy and the self. *Policy and Politics, 45*(2), 121–136.

Wilkinson, R. & Pickett, K. (2010). *The spirit level: Why equality is better for everyone.* Penguin.

Wulf, W. (1989, March). The National Collaboratory. In *Towards a national collaboratory.* Unpublished report of a National Science Foundation invitational workshop. Rockefeller University, New York.

Wulf, W. (1993). The collaboratory opportunity. *Science, 261*, 854–855.

Zielke, J. (2019). Dwelling: On the design, implementation and analysis of 'story houses' as multi-modal research method. *Qualitative Research in Psychology.* https://doi.org/10.1080/14780887.2019.1677834

Chapter 6

Coproduction and care planning

Catherine Mills

This chapter focuses on coproduction and the care planning process in mental health settings. It tracks the evolution of care planning over time and introduces some of the barriers and facilitators to good care planning as experienced in different settings: a female acute ward, a ward for people with dementia and a secure setting, all within Mersey Care NHS Foundation Trust (MCNHSFT). My own interest in care planning stems from two sources: first, my professional background in general nursing, and second, my experience as a user of mental health services, spanning a period of around 40 years.

In mental health services, care planning has historically been a professional endeavour, based on a medical model of treatment, with practitioner-led assessments and wholly organised around professional judgements of problems and needs, with interventions designed accordingly. Within such a traditional approach, the service user is a passive recipient of professional interest and attention. Recently, with growing interest in notions of individual agency and personal recovery, there is much more of an expectation that service users become active participants in their own care. Care planning thus becomes an area of professional practice where service users can become empowered by offering their insights as to how they see their future and how they might achieve their aspirations. For example, they may have career ambitions they wish to pursue, or they may wish to take up a hobby or voluntary activity. They may share insights into how their medication is affecting them that informs their treatment plan. This all helps create a mutually respectful, coproduced care plan that the service user feels ownership of.

Thus, care planning has been evolving, and these days mental health services that want service users to actively engage with them are adopting a coproduction approach. We can see it in local contracts, research and service design. The New Economics Foundation (Slay & Penny, 2014) defines coproduction as:

> ... a relationship where professionals and citizens share power to design, plan and deliver support together, recognising that both partners have vital contributions to make in order to improve quality of life for people and communities [...] it is the most effective method of achieving outcomes with people. (p.7)

From this perspective, coproduction starts from the belief that everyone is equal, and no one should hold power over another. Everyone has something of value to contribute to the process.

Coproducing care plans in unlikely places

Albert Dzur (2019) highlights the achievements of certain professionals in managing to facilitate coproduction in services and settings that, at first sight, appear unpromising settings for such an endeavour. One such setting might be assumed to be mental health services, where the operation of mental health legislation and other risk management considerations pose potential barriers to effective and authentic coproduction. Nevertheless, the examples presented in this chapter show that successes in coproduction can, indeed, be achieved in the most unlikely places. Furthermore, it is arguably the case that not to attempt coproduction, regardless of prevailing impediments, is a failure of professionalism and could in many respects be counterproductive with respect to anxieties about risk and safety.

So, what are the dangers of failing to coproduce? Chambers and colleagues (2014) highlight how people detained under the Mental Health Act are typically denied the ability to contribute to the decision-making process about their care plan. The consequence of this can be a sense of powerlessness and helplessness, which can have a detrimental impact on their recovery. Coercive interventions become the order of the day. Service users lacking dignity can literally lose their will to live (Chockinov, 2012). Services characterised by conflict and restrictive practices find that the potential to establish therapeutic engagement and alliances is constrained (Cleary, 2004; Gilburt, et al., 2008; Quirk & Lelliott, 2001).

In such circumstances, the sort of co-operative and democratic processes necessary for effective care coproduction are likely to be undermined. Coercive services become stressful and injurious places for staff to work in, so professionals and service users both have a stake in working towards more peaceful care environments. Chambers and colleagues (2014) suggest it is possible for the frequency and impact of violence and conflict in acute mental health settings to be reduced by the use of advance directives as part of the care programme/care planning process. Numerous other researchers have shown that efforts to minimise the use of restrictive practices also result in improved ward atmosphere and better relationships. These successes often involve working with staff to enhance co-operative aspects of care (Bowers et al., 2015; Duxbury et al., 2019; Huckshorn, 2004).

Care planning and the Care Programme Approach

Contemporary mental healthcare in the UK became organised according to case management principles and structures in the early 1990s. This was framed by a Care Programme Approach (CPA) policy (Department of Health, 2001), which still operates, with modifications. The devolved nations (Scotland, Wales and Northern Ireland) have taken slightly different approaches but remain committed to care co-ordination. The CPA was introduced in 1991 and the original guidance was updated in 1999. It is designed to ensure that care provision is service user focused and driven. There are eight domains that a relevant care plan should include:

- mental health
- diet
- medication and side effects
- discharge planning
- physical health
- behavioural support
- risk planning/safety
- inpatient leave plan.

Hannigan and colleagues (2018) discuss how care co-ordination is central to the care planning process to ensure that needs are met and integrated services are provided. They conclude that care co-ordination is not consistently being done in the way policymakers expected or imagined. Coffey and colleagues (2017) state that the terms 'care co-ordination' and 'care planning' are often used interchangeably, yet they imply different sets of processes, practices and experiences for people working in and using services.[1] Co-operatively involving service users in the construction of care plans could be a prime example of coproduction in practice, and such processes of care planning represent substantial opportunities to enact policy goals regarding personalised care and recovery (Coffey et al., 2019).

Care plans are audited and inspected by national bodies. The regulator, the Care Quality Commission (2013), has noted 'a significant gap between the realities observed in practice and the ambitions of the national mental health policy' (p.5). With the emphasis on targets, this can come at the expense of the relational aspects of care planning. One example is the target of ensuring that 95% of care plans are signed by the service user, while neglecting to assess if care plans are coproduced and actually delivered (Department of Health, 2001).

Risk planning and safety are central to the care planning process and this can be considered with regard to: a) the risk the person presents to themselves in the form of suicide or vulnerability, and b) the risk the person may present to others (with the former being the most common risk identified). According to Coffey and colleagues (2016), it appears that risk is the least likely topic for authentic coproduction. These authors suggest that, although the picture is not universally negative, four times more people reported not being involved in their risk assessments than those providing a more positive account. Below is a quote taken from a research interview with a family member in one English NHS site, who felt they had been left out of the care planning process and, paradoxically, also felt left to manage safety and risk by themselves:

Interviewer: 'Do you feel your safety and the safety of (patient's name) have been considered in their care planning and co-ordination?'

Respondent: 'No, definitely not, 100% no way. I've stopped her cutting herself loads of times, I've stopped her taking overdoses, I've had to hide tablets, all sorts of stuff… nothing's been discussed with me.'

Mersey Care: A modern mental health service provider

Service users under the care of MCNHSFT, a secondary healthcare service, will either receive standard care or care under CPA. Those under standard care will have more straightforward needs and contact with fewer agencies. Those under CPA will have more complex needs, perhaps involving contact with multiple agencies and presenting with a higher degree of risk. All new service

---

1. Care co-ordination is the process whereby the inputs of different members of the care team are strategically organised and delivered. They all should be working to the care plan that, under CPA, also ought to indicate who is responsible for which aspects of the plan.

users undergo a full assessment of need before determining whether they are cared for under CPA or non-CPA (standard care). All service users subject to CPA will have an allocated care co-ordinator. Sometimes service users may be acutely distressed and unwell, or their mental capacity may be compromised, in which case it is particularly important to draw on the resources of the wider family or independent advocacy services (Newbigging et al., 2015). Various settings within MCNHSFT have offered different possibilities for developing coproduction practices relating to care planning. I now turn to consider three distinct examples of these.

Care planning and coproduction on an acute mental health ward for women

The care planning model used is based around the domains discussed above.

On the acute ward, the named nurse and the service user are jointly responsible for updating the care plan on a weekly basis. The named nurse will usually be a registered nurse. Care plans are recorded in the clinical notes so they can be shared with the care team.

Historically, the women have engaged well with coproducing the care plan, the only exception being if they are acutely unwell. The weekly multidisciplinary team meeting informs the care plan. Families are invited to this meeting, with the consent of the service user. Unfortunately, when in the initial acute stage of illness, the service user may not want the family to be involved as they may see them as being responsible for their being sectioned. Often this resolves itself as recovery takes place.

Some patients are admitted and detained under the Mental Health Act and are extremely unhappy with the service that has 'sectioned' them, and consequently do not want to spend time with nursing staff. In this instance, the nursing staff will take information initially from the family, care co-ordinator and the clinical information system, while persevering to establish a relationship.

A further barrier to good coproduced care planning is that the named nurse system requires an allocation of time to the care planning process. Usually this is one hour. However, the nurses did not always have this time available, owing to other pressures, such as medication rounds, reviews, administration and so on. They reported that not actually having the time to sit down with the service user was often a barrier.

Care planning and coproduction on a ward for people with dementia

Before admission to this ward, a pre-identification of need is carried out. Admissions usually happen as a result of a referral from a consultant or community nurse. Information is also gained from the service user's wider support network. While some service users have the mental capacity to contribute towards the initial assessment, often this is not the case, because of the level of dementia experienced by the service user. To maximise the service user contribution, staff will write things down and use pictures to try to achieve effective communication.

It is important to gather information about the service user's likes and dislikes, sleeping patterns and aspects of daily living where support may be required. The ward has an assistant practitioner who assesses the service user's physical presentation and actively monitors this.

One means by which staff facilitate communication with the service user is by life-story work. Here the staff work with the service user and, where appropriate, the family to explore their history and interests. These give staff a reference point by which they can relate to the service user and stimulate communication, thereby offering insights into personal preferences and providing the basis for care planning discussions.

In terms of care planning, where there is scope to involve the service user in coproducing the care plan, this happens. Where the service user lacks capacity, the family are invited to contribute to the care plan. Within dementia services, the family are essential to the care planning process and an important source of information. Advocacy services can also be called on to support the service user and help them contribute to the care plan. This may be particularly important if the service user does not have any family.

Care planning in secure services

The decision to admit to a secure service will be based on a comprehensive risk assessment and detailed consideration of how the risks identified can be safely managed while in hospital. Mersey Care is one of only three trusts in England that provide the whole range of mental health services across different levels of security, including low-, medium- and high-secure facilities. Forensic mental healthcare deals with individuals who pose a severe risk to others and often present with significant management problems within hospital settings. The care of such individuals creates a tension with regard to balancing care and safety, and between protecting the interests of the patients and those of wider society.

In keeping with the Mental Health Act 1983 Code of Practice (Department of Health, 2015), MCNHSFT states that 'patients should be given the opportunity to be involved in planning, developing and reviewing their own care and treatment'.

The basis of every nursing care plan is to assess, plan, implement and evaluate. Everything within the nursing care plan should be based on SMART (Specific, Measurable, Achievable, Realistic and Time-bound) principles.

In MCNHSFT secure services, the patient must always be included when constructing the care plan. It should be written in the first person, in language that is clear and easy to understand. It should be dated and have a positive, socially-orientated approach to care. The care plan is produced collaboratively and coproductively, based on the three conversations of past, self and future. Even patients who challenge the system may be amenable to co-operation for long periods, so it is important to look for patient strengths. The care plans in secure services are reviewed by the named nurse on a monthly basis and the patient is offered a copy of the care plan. The nursing care plan must guide the work of other team members and support quality, continuity of care, risk management and communication.

Relationships are central to secure nursing (see Chapter 3) and are pivotal in creating opportunities for people to behave appropriately, with a view to eventually being able to return to society. In situations that become extreme, staff are required to personalise care and their own role within it, showing they are human, as this is necessary both from a recovery and a security perspective. Staff need to understand what is going on for the patient and build up trust so they can gain important information that the care team rely on. All this needs to be achieved while, at the same time, maintaining professional boundaries with patients. McKeown and colleagues (2016) discuss the juxtaposition of mental health services in a secure setting with offender rehabilitation goals and suggest that the aim of recovery could be to achieve a meaningful life. The balance between therapy and security is crucial. They advocate a 'third way' approach to care planning whereby the recovery-orientation approach, which wishes to see the best in people, is considered alongside the forensic culture, which recognises potential for the worst in people and seeks to contain this. McKeown and colleagues acknowledge the complexities of this client group and that patients may work to escape the identity of serious offender or killer, and how this may be associated with expressions of regret and remorse that, in turn, can form the basis for co-operative dialogue relating to the person's care plan.

All patients in secure services are subject to the full CPA, and the nursing care plan needs to inform and link with this. The nursing care plan is influenced by trauma-informed care, where the emphasis is on the patient from childhood, not exclusively the index offence. Wall and colleagues (2016) define this as:

> ... a framework for human service delivery that is based on a knowledge and understanding of how trauma affects people's lives, their service needs and service usage. (p.9)

In high-secure settings people often present with complex behaviours related to past trauma.

Proctor and colleagues (2017) identify several factors in inpatient units that can be retraumatising for patients or insensitive to their trauma history:

- safety
- trustworthiness and transparency
- peer support
- collaboration and mutuality
- empowerment, voice and choice
- cultural, historical and gender issues.

Improving sensitivity must include appreciation of the importance of the physical and social environment. Services may invalidate a patient's experience, thereby reinforcing maladaptive behaviours and coping skills.

The use of seclusion and restraint is one practice that can cause distress and aggression and re-traumatise the individual. This can destabilise the care, treatment and therapeutic alliance between the patient and staff. Trauma-informed care has emerged as a critical consideration in prioritising treatment and service delivery. It is likely to result in both short- and long-term cost effectiveness (Quadara, 2015). In high-secure settings, there is a small number of individuals who are cared for in what effectively amounts to long-term seclusion, segregated from free association with other patients. Specialist staff try to facilitate processes analogous to 'decompression', whereby these people can gradually return to the mainstream community (Mason et al., 1996). This is very much a communicative endeavour, with features of coproduction evident. It shows how, even in the most extreme circumstances, some degree of trust, co-operation and democratic engagement can be possible, if very difficult to achieve.

In these environments, the notion of recovery is complicated by aspects of mental health, desistance from violence or other offending, and consensus on what it means to return to a good life. Discussions on this territory can be fraught with emotive hazards and interpersonal sensitivities. They can be hard work for all concerned. The nursing care plan must embrace a recovery-orientated approach that reflects this, and certain recovery-orientated principles are to be observed. These recovery-orientated principles include the following:

- Often there is no good way to reframe the past, so talk about the future, not the past.

- Talk about the patient's ideas of success and how to get there.
- Always write in the first person.
- Treat the person as they could be, not necessarily as they are.
- Look for hope, encourage it and,. where the person loses hope, report it immediately.
- Be positive.
- Always be sincere and genuine.
- Always seek the patient view and record quotes if possible.
- Always be honest.
- Always complete a Recovery Star[2] for every CPA or significant clinical change.

Care plans in secure services need to fulfil safety criteria and caring needs. Care plans are currently audited remotely by random checks. Patients are asked about their knowledge of care plans and checks are made to ensure they have been offered copies of their care plan. The aim in secure services is to have the care plan accessible via a laptop that is safe for patients to access. Within secure services, MCNHSFT is also developing their own bespoke Recovery Star.

Family engagement in the care planning process tends to be variable and inconsistent. With the high-secure hospital receiving patients from all over England and Wales, it can be logistically challenging to involve families. In the experience of secure service staff, families often are not interested in participating in care plans, and sometimes the patients do not want their family to be involved. However, this can result from a lack of appropriate support and facilities to enable more consistent engagement with and involvement of families. MCNHSFT has invested in a dedicated co-ordinator for such family involvement, which has led to various developments in the high-secure setting, including provision of information, a support group for families, bespoke events, improvements to visiting arrangements and a visitor centre. This support for families featured as a good practice example in a national toolkit produced by NHS England.[3]

McKeown and colleagues (2019) concur that providing institutional support can enable families to cope with the additional pressures that arise from supporting a family member with both serious mental health needs and

---

2. The Recovery Star is a format for assessment of recovery across a number of different dimensions, represented diagrammatically by the points of a star, and allowing for self and staff rating of progress in each domain (see Dickens et al., 2012).

3. www.england.nhs.uk/wp-content/uploads/2018/05/secure-carers-toolkit-v2.pdf

involvement in criminal offending – a doubly stigmatising perspective. This is needed to increase their coping skills, improve communication and enhance their knowledge about mental healthcare and treatment options. Furthermore, well-supported and engaged families can then become a valuable ally to professional care providers, contributing to care planning in a 'triangle of care'. *Triangle of Care* (Carers Trust, 2013) is guidance that sets out a range of challenges for engaging carers and family members in the care planning process. It requires that services include the carer in the assessment, treatment and care planning process and reinforces the importance of the relationship between the service, the patient and the carer. Only when there is full triangulation can service user experience be optimised and everyone's needs truly be met.

Where a patient does not consent to sharing information with the carer, it can be all too easy for the staff to cite 'confidentiality' as a barrier to involving families. However, as highlighted in *Triangle of Care* (Carers Trust, 2013), if a patient does not consent to share, there is nothing to stop the service listening to the carer and gathering vital information or providing generic support for carers. Staff can, for example, listen to carers' concerns and offer general information and advice.

Psychosocial interventions with families can help repair relationships that have broken down and improve communication within families, for everyone's benefit. This, and other forms of family support and involvement, can thus be important and promote helpful partnership working with care teams, with a positive impact on active co-operation with ongoing care and treatment. Individuals and families who are participants in care planning are more likely to actively support resultant plans, and this decreases the chance of patient relapse, reduces distress in the family, and improves interaction between patient and family.

Coproduction can present challenges to both staff and patients. Care planning has historically focused on professional identification of patients' problems and keeping people safe. This traditional approach was satisfied with unreflective compliance with treatment, but the outcome could often actually be poor co-operation or outright resistance. Sometimes staff attitudes take time to shift to a more collaborative, relationship-based model of care planning. When working coproductively with patients who are serious offenders, it is important not to let them down and to ensure that honesty underpins the whole care planning process. Interestingly, when service users in secure settings are more thoroughly involved in care planning and other decision-making, they usually appreciate the process, becoming more co-operative generally, even in circumstances where they do not immediately get what they are asking for (McKeown et al., 2014).

Conclusions

MCNHSFT and other NHS organisations aspire to meet the standards stipulated in *Triangle of Care* (2013). From the three examples outlined above, we can see that services do endeavour to engage carers and family members, although, from my personal experience of working with wards and teams, the standards achieved can be variable. As with trying to find the time to sit down with the patient to coproduce care plans, it can be challenging to arrange to meet formally with family carers to listen to their story and gather information regarding a patient's needs and their own. Staff working in various ward environments have multiple demands on their time, including substantial administrative burdens, and we must strive to ensure that direct patient contact is not compromised. That said, it should not be ignored that the process of involvement in coproductive care planning has its own positive impacts.

We recognise that risk (to self and others) and security need to be balanced with the therapeutic approach and that risk is an area where coproduction can be absent. Risk challenges services in their quest to keep the patient and public safe and interacts with broader forces within an increasingly risk-averse society.

I think it is fair to say that, along with national developments, MCNHSFT and other organisations have come a long way in striving to genuinely coproduce care plans with patients. However, it is a constant challenge to identify time to ensure this happens consistently and to involve families and carers in the process. The benefits to patients and carers have been identified in the examples described in the three settings above. Coproduction is undoubtedly the way forward and a journey on which MCNHSFT and other service providers are fully engaged. There is, of course, always room for further improvement, and dynamic leadership will be required if the democratic demands of more radical and impatient voices are to be met.

References

Bowers, L., James, K., Quirk, A., Simpson, A., Stewart, D. & Hodsoll, J. (2015). Reducing conflict and containment rates on acute psychiatric wards: The Safewards cluster randomised controlled trial. *International Journal of Nursing Studies, 52*(9), 1412–1422.

Care Quality Commission. (2013). *Monitoring the Mental Health Act in 2011/12*. Care Quality Commission.

Carers Trust (2013). Triangle of care: A guide to best practice in mental health care in England (2nd ed.). Carers Trust.

Chambers, M., Gallagher, A., Borschmann, R., Gillard, S., Turner, K. & Kantaris, X. (2014). The experiences of detained mental health service users: Issues of dignity in care. *BMC Medical Ethics, 15*(50), 1–8.

Chockinov, H.M. (2012). *Dignity therapy: Final words for final days.* Oxford University Press.

Cleary, M. (2004). The realities of mental health nursing in acute inpatient environments. *International Journal of Mental Health Nursing, 13*(1), 53–60.

Coffey, M., Cohen, R., Faulkner, A., Hannigan, B., Simpson, A & Barlow, S. (2016). Ordinary risks and accepted fictions: How contrasting and competing priorities work in risk assessment and mental health care planning. *Health Expectations, 20*(3), 471–483.

Coffey, M., Hannigan, B. & Simpson, A. (2017). Care planning and co-ordination: Imperfect solutions in an imperfect world. *Journal of Psychiatric and Mental Health Nursing, 24*(6), 333–334.

Coffey, M., Hannigan, B., Barlow, S., Cartwright, M., Cohen, R., Faulkner, A., Jones, A. & Simpson, A. (2019). Recovery-focused mental health care planning and co-ordination in acute inpatient mental health settings: A cross national comparative mixed methods study. *BMC Psychiatry, 19*(1), 115. https://doi: 10.1186/s12888-019-2094-7

Department of Health. (2001). *An audit pack for monitoring the Care Programme Approach.* Department of Health.

Department of Health. (2015). *Mental Health Act 1983: Code of practice.* Department of Health. https://assets.publishing.service.gov.uk/government/uploads/system/uploads/attachment_data/file/435512/MHA_Code_of_Practice.PDF

Dickens, G., Weleminsky, J., Onifade, Y. & Sugarman, P. (2012). Recovery star: Validating user recovery. *The Psychiatrist, 36*(2), 45–50.

Duxbury, J., Baker, J., Downe, S., Jones, F., Greenwood, P., Thygesen, H., McKeown, M., Price, O., Scholes, A., Thomson, G. & Whittington, R. (2019). Minimising the use of physical restraint in acute mental health services: The outcome of a restraint reduction programme ('REsTRAIN YOURSELF'). *International Journal of Nursing Studies, 95*, 40–48.

Dzur A.W. (2019). *Democracy inside: Participatory innovation in unlikely places.* Oxford University Press.

Gilburt, H., Rose, D. & Slade, M. (2008). The importance of relationships in mental health care: A qualitative study of service users' experiences of psychiatric hospital admission in the UK. *BMC Health Services Research, 8*(1), 92.

Hannigan, B., Simpson, A., Coffey, M., Barlow, S. & Jones, A. (2018). Care co-ordination as imagined, care co-ordination as done: Findings from a cross-national mental health systems study. *International Journal of Integrated Care, 18*(3), 12. doi: 10.5334/ijic.3978

Huckshorn, K.A. (2004). Reducing seclusion and restraint use in mental health settings: Core strategies for prevention. *Journal of Psychosocial Nursing and Mental Health Services, 42*(9), 22–33.

Mason, T., Henighen, M., Chandley, M. & Johnson, D. (1996). Decompression from long-term seclusion. *Psychiatric Care, 3*(6), 217–225.

McKeown, M., Jones, F., Foy, P., Wright, K., Paxton, T. & Blackmon, M. (2016). Looking back, looking forward: Recovery journeys in a high secure hospital. *International Journal of Mental Health Nursing, 25*, 234–242.

McKeown, M., Jones, F., Stewart, S. & Foster, S. (2019). Family support and involvement in secure mental health services. In N. Evans (Ed.), *Family work in mental health: A skills approach* (pp.83–102). M&K.

McKeown, M., Jones, F., Wright, K., Spandler, H., Wright, J., Fletcher, H., Duxbury, J., McVittie, J., Simon & Turton, W. (2014). It's the talk: A study of involvement practices in secure mental health services. *Health Expectations, 19*(3), 570–579.

Newbigging, K., Ridley, J., McKeown, M., Poursanidou, K., Able, L., Machin, K., Cruse, K. & Sadd, J. (2015). *Independent mental health advocacy – The right to be heard: The practice and context of professional advocacy in mental health services.* Jessica Kingsley.

Proctor, N., Ayling B., Croft, L., DeGaris, P., Devine, M., Dimanic, A., Di Fiore, L, Eaton, H., Edwards, M., Ferguson, M., Lang, S., Rebellato, A., Shaw K. & Sullivan, R. (2017). *Trauma-informed approaches in forensic mental health: A practical resource for health professionals.* University of South Australia.

Quadara, A. (2015). *Implementing trauma-informed systems of care in health settings: The WITH study.* State of Knowledge paper. Australian Institute of Family Studies.

Quirk, A. & Lelliott, P. (2001). What do we know about life on acute psychiatric wards in the UK? A review of the research evidence. *Social Science & Medicine, 53*(12), 1565–1574.

Slay, J. & Penny, J. (2014). *Commissioning for outcomes and co-production: A practical guide for local authorities.* New Economics Foundation.

Wall. L., Higgins. D. & Hunter, C. (2016). *Trauma informed care in child/family welfare services.* CFCA paper, no. 37. Australian Institute of Family studies. https://aifs.gov.au/cfca/publications/trauma-informed-care-child-family-welfare-services/introduction

Chapter 7

Coproduction and addiction

Lucy Webb and Amanda Clayson

Picture this: an education charity sets up a primary school in a remote rural district in sub-Saharan Africa. The school is well stocked with books, desks, a blackboard and a teacher. The villagers are all invited to send their children to the school. Local elders are told the children will learn to read, write and be good at numbers and will be able to get a job when they are older. A few children turn up the first day. The next day, a few more, but slowly the numbers of attendees drop off. Soon, there are no children attending the school. Efforts are made to encourage the parents to send their children to the school. Discussions are held with village elders. The children are offered free uniforms, school meals, books to take home. The children return, eat the meals, take the books and disappear.

This is a real scenario currently playing out in the Namibian Kalahari, where the San people live. The school is now mostly populated by children of the pastoral tribe of the area, the Herero, and the San children are nowhere to be seen. Clearly, the San people do not value what this school offers, and the children are more usually found honing their remarkable skills in tracking, hunting and surviving in the Kalahari Desert, as the hunter-gatherers they have always been.

So, what has this to do with coproduction? In this chapter we want to focus on how coproduction challenges people to confront and understand prejudices in values, beliefs and lifestyles – their own and others' – and develop mutual understanding to work together to solve shared problems. To do this, we will make use of our experience of working with people with very different values and lifestyles that often present service providers with the barriers of incompatible values: people with problems with drug or alcohol. The inclusion of global development examples is more meaningful here than simply providing an analogy. What we have learned about coproduction with reluctant partners is that the economic and environmental sciences have already applied coproduction principles to partnership working and have discovered much that the health and social care sciences can use when challenged by multiple barriers (Arnstein, 1969).

Addiction as a health and social care problem has often presented a challenge to service providers and policymakers, especially when using a hierarchical, medical approach. Treatment for substance use problems works. There is plenty evidence to show that, once someone with a substance use problem engages and maintains contact with substance misuse services, there is a high probability that they will become abstinent and, in the longer term, maintain a healthier lifestyle (Gossop, 2006; Public Health England, 2017). And there's the problem: engaging someone in treatment, whether it is for substance misuse or a mental health issue, presents services with the task of bridging the gap of mistrust, stigmatisation and self-doubt that has alienated many people in the first place.

Arguably, coproduced health services for, say, hospice provision, emergency services and outpatient clinics is a challenge, but it is often easy to engage service users, family members and interested members of the public in a forum to discuss and plan together. It is an easy sell because it is in everyone's interest. But, like our San people above, if there is not a shared goal... well, you can lead a horse to water...

At risk of labelling problematic substance users as socially excluded, recent history of service provision suggests that this population faces barriers to engagement with treatment services (EMCDDA, 2003). The history of drug policy in the UK contributes to this mistrust. After all, drug use is linked to criminality, social exclusion (i.e. homelessness, imprisonment) and stigmatisation (Public Health England, 2017; UK Drug Policy Commission, 2010). Just think what the 2008 UK anti-drugs campaign 'Rat on a Rat' did to alienate drug users. The campaign consisted of pictures of rats and a slogan 'Drug dealers ruin lives'. There were even rewards offered to the public to report a drug dealer. The reality of addiction to drugs is, of course, that there is little or no distinction between a 'user' and a 'dealer'; giving a mate a wrap of heroin when they need it is dealing in the eyes of the law; becoming a supplier to your network of friends secures your own supply of heroin.

Our experience of working coproductively with people with substance use problems has helped us explore what coproduction is, or should be; what the challenges are in working with potentially reluctant partners, and what we have found useful in modelling our approach. In this chapter, we will outline the experiences of working coproductively with communities where substance use is a defining issue and attempt to share the knowledge and understanding gained from the many clash points we have encountered. Typically, these have been the times when we have learned the most.

This chapter draws on the reflections from the perspectives of a community partner (Amanda Clayson) and an academic partner (Lucy Webb), and the voices of our community partners. From our very early experience of different cultural worlds, the process has enabled us to reframe our different roles and strengths. We want to outline our learning of what has 'worked' for everyone, but also what we have found unhelpful or downright obstructive.

Background to our work

Since 2013, we have been engaged in a series of activities collectively titled Recovery Voice in Action. This was an exploration of the meaning of recovery as understood and expressed by people in recovery from problems with alcohol or other drugs. It involved many contact points and activities, including the Manchester Recovery Walk in 2014, coproductive research and promotion activities that used media-supported technology – and just plain socialising.

Coproduction origins and uses

The diverse origins and strands of coproduction and its context-driven principles make it hard to define in its application, but the fundamental driver is the need for mutual consultation and decision-making, based on a sharing of knowledge and values. A philosophy underpinning coproduction as a tool for governance derives from the work of economist Elinor Ostrom and colleagues, who identified that end users of services have no say in service planning and delivery (Ostrom & Baugh, 1973). Such top-down service provision takes no account of the inherent assets, knowledge and skills within the community, and disempowers community members and populations. Economists such as Cahn and Goodwin (Cahn, 2001; Goodwin et al., 2003) proposed applying coproduction through economic exchange, such as time banking, which recognises and values what non-fiscal community contributions bring to local economies. These early ideas of resource exchange have developed into models of collaborative working across many fields of governance, particularly environmental collaboration (e.g. Berkes, 2010).

It is now the norm for environmental management projects to work in partnership with indigenous and local populations to preserve the natural environment. The San people in the introduction are now a vital part of conservation in the Kalahari. Who better to be the government's eyes and ears to reduce poaching and monitor the flora and fauna than the people with the skills to do so and knowledge of the area?

Coproduction has morphed from bottom-up economic and environmental management to citizen inclusion in health and social care planning (Glynos & Speed, 2012), with UK health policy adopting a 'citizen consumer' approach, ensuring end users of services and the community are involved in commissioning, prioritising and collaborating in health research (Shippee et al., 2013). Coproduction is recognised as economically cost-effective (Horne et al., 2013); it improves service planning, local representation, the adoption of local knowledge and 'buy in' of community members (Coote, 2002; Needham & Carr, 2009). Durose and colleagues (2011) suggest it has become a vehicle for social justice, enabling democratic knowledge production and grassroots representation. In this way, it reduces the power differential between the expert and the layperson.

Coproduced research

The key principles of coproduction research are the reduction of the power differential between partners, and equal exchange of knowledge. In research, this means recognising and valuing the assets and strengths of end users, addressing whole-person (and community) contexts and adopting holistic approaches to solutions (Boyle et al., 2010). There is growing use of research approaches that attempt to be inclusive of everyone who is involved in the research process and its outcomes. Participatory research, for example, ensures that everyone, including those being researched, has a meaningful say in the process. This should mean that even the question being researched is identified by all stakeholders as being important (Asaba & Suarez-Balcazar, 2018).

This approach converges with the growth of asset-based and mutual aid principles of addiction recovery in the UK. Recovery as a social movement refocuses the problem-solving lens towards wellbeing, quality of life and community engagement, as well as sobriety (Best & Laudet, 2010). Importantly, recovery as a social movement focuses on mutual aid, with communities of people in recovery finding their own collective assets and values, and breaking away from the stigmatising focus on disease model definitions of addiction (White, 2007).

For Boyle and colleagues (2010), coproduction demonstrates specific features of recognising and enhancing people as assets, working equally and in partnership (mutuality and reciprocity), working with peer support networks, and having integrated partnership working between different agents (blurring distinctions). For the academic or professional partner, the role should be one of facilitating rather than leading or delivering. The research programme partners for the UK's Economic and Social Research Council (ESRC) N8 Research Partnership describe coproduction as a meta-methodology – an overarching research approach in which boundaries between pure and applied research are blurred, and a process that confers public benefits beyond academia or professional practice (N8/ESRC, 2016). For the N8/ESRC research programme, coproduction research should strive for academic excellence but at the same time present flexible working between partners and produce inclusive and actionable evidence.

This way of working presents challenges, and these typically will involve time commitment, especially for community members; inflexibility of organisational administration processes; ethical procedures, and financial management (N8/ESRC, 2016). While these elements of research processes have tried-and-tested procedures in traditional research, they present a challenge to coproductive methodologies that often require removal of 'traditional' ways of working and a major shift in thinking to meet their principles of equality and value.

The mutuality and reciprocity principle of coproduction suggests, for Boyle and colleagues (2010), a sharing of responsibility and expectancies and, as expressed by Wehrens (2014), an interdependent flow of knowledge, in which partners are not seen as existing in separate, rigid domains, and where boundaries can be negotiated and are flexible. To adhere to this principle, the research process needs to involve all partners equally so that recognition of the need for research, the research question and project planning are as much driven by the community members as by professional researchers or policymakers.

Our project

The Recovery Voice in Action project was led by the VoiceBox community team and community groups, and included academic partners, with the aim of exploring the experience of recovery and to support mutual aid social recovery links and activities.

Many of the activities consisted of a series of community-based recovery outreach and showcasing events, which included participant-controlled structured interviewing via video. People interviewed were both event attendees and the 'crew' themselves.

VoiceBox

VoiceBox is a participant-controlled, computer-assisted interviewing tool and the accompanying community organisation (the 'crew'). It facilitates data collection via structured interviews or 'voxpop' commentary (Cox et al., 2016). A key aspect of this project was the incorporation of people in recovery as VoiceBox 'crew', design consultants, recruiters/outreach, interviewers and data interpreters. The research project was part of a wider community project of involvement and engagement, consisting of a loose affiliation of community recovery members around the VoiceBox crew, community liaison and academic facilitators.

Collecting reflections

We collected data from these projects from multiple sources, including The Brink, a dry bar in Liverpool run by a national drug and alcohol service. The evaluation gathered a range of digital assets, including film, photography and audio recordings. After completion of the evaluation, a group of participants and VoiceBox continued working together, forming the Voices from the Brink community research crew to explore the value of the digital assets to develop better understanding of the meaning of recovery. Data were collected by all three partners over the three-year period (2013–2016), in the form of individual and group reflections gathered in written and digital formats, including film and audio recordings.

The projects afforded opportunities for all partners to discuss methods of working and identify barriers and problem-solve, while exploring and testing the principles of coproduction.

Project analysis examined the reflections, contexts of data collection and impact on each of the three partners. From this came the R Factor: a framework with which to chart and identify factors inherent in the coproduction process when researchers and community members inhabit different values spaces and world views.

The R Factor Framework

Reach

A key factor from the outset was that the learning from activity would 'touch' a wider group of people than would normally have access to 'traditional' research outlets. Channels of communication and research translation became embedded in the coproductive process; snowballing became commonplace, as working through recovery communities and networks (face-to-face and virtual) facilitated getting very close to the issues through the people experiencing them:

> This research means something to us – it's grounded in who we are and what we know - we want people to hear about it and to learn from it – me taking this to the services and groups that I know or talking to others and getting them to talk about it is important to me – I want to get this out there. (Community researcher)

Reason

Our findings highlighted that reasons for initial and ongoing participation varied considerably for different people and changed over time. For community researchers (with lived experience), the fundamental reason was predominantly to promote recovery and help others. This proved to be a positive factor in sustaining the research process and 'pushing' for the activity to be extended wider than the original focus. It was not the intention to negate personal motivations of academics to improve experiences of people impacted by substance use, but the agenda was inevitably linked to their university role and the need to demonstrate research activity. It was also clear that research activity goals are often governed by the funder. During the life of the project, some funding was accessed, but most community researchers had no external resources. This led to different outcome expectations. Where funding was secured, traditional research outcomes (practice recommendations, reporting, dissemination) continued to be used as benchmarks for success and completion of the research activity, with funders' expectations privileged over community needs and goals. Although a lack of funding presented significant barriers for community partners, it afforded a level of flexibility and 'freedom' to enable them to allow the research agenda to 'unfold'. Overall, the sense was that the challenges and implications were poorly understood organisationally, which often led to tokenistic support.

Reciprocity

The sharing of knowledge was, arguably, easier for the academic members than for the partners, and this illustrated an issue particularly when working with communities in which low self-esteem and stigmatisation are barriers to inclusion. Although community partners initially struggled to acknowledge their power in the knowledge and its value to the research, there was a clear shift over time as a coproductive culture 'bedded in'.

Power is also inherent in research language and processes in that, essentially, coproduced research is still research and can have too much organisational reliance on academic processes. In order to meet the needs for research excellence, there remains currently a need to either identify the equivalents of methodological rigour (i.e. respondent validation) or emphasise the particular strengths of coproduction, such as authenticity and applicability.

Recovery

The process of being involved in research made a positive contribution to people's recovery. This included their understanding of themselves as people, and as people in recovery. Many examples pointed to individuals' self-learning, the impact of sharing of experiences and the self-esteem that came with being genuine partners in the research.

> What comes up for me is the level of growth, for me personally and for others in the Crew. When we first talked about the idea of research, I thought it was something that universities did and came and asked questions […] I wasn't long out of treatment and my recovery was my priority, not talking to people about research. I know now that it's not like that. Being part of this has been part of my recovery […] I'm a researcher in my own life and helping others in similar situations to me […] that's so good for my recovery. (Member of the VoiceBox crew)

Relationship

This area was the one that had the most impact for all of the partners. The growing relationship between each of the participants was crucial to the whole approach to delivering something that had to be genuinely coproduced. Relationships formed and were based on a real and deep understanding of each other as individuals and their positions and experiences (academic and lived). It allowed all parties to take risks and created a richer dialogue and led to the robustness of the curation and understanding.

Reward

The principles of coproduction emphasise the need for everyone to benefit from the involvement. It was important that all partners acknowledged and shared what the benefit was for them. These rewards were naturally different and reflected the reasons partners wanted to be involved. In recovery from addiction, a key 'reward' appeared to be enacting the principles of recovery through helping others, combating stigmatisation, and self-representation (speaking truth to power). Other types of 'reward' included the perceived 'credibility' of being associated with a higher education institution and engaged on 'proper' research. Although this was identified as a positive outcome, it also stimulated feelings of 'rub' where the perceived status of each partner was different.

Risk

This included the perceived risk of the co-productive process and associated power relationship:

> I noticed I got panicky thinking that we had to be doing this and this, otherwise the funders get upset and the university management gets upset. It felt 'risky' to be letting go of this control and allow other

people to take over. Even talking about it in this way just shows how the traditional research relationship starts getting into a power relationship. (Academic researcher)

Robustness

Here the concern was always around how much the research would be seen as robust in traditional research terms – for example, having a research question in mind that could be tested through well-established research approaches in data collection and analysis. What we found was the robustness came from the authenticity of the data collected by being able to get 'up close and personal', which was a key benefit of the coproductive research process, allowing us to reframe what we meant by 'robust'. By using each person's experiences as a resource, the whole process was more robust as there were more checks and balances, in particular in relation to the authenticity of the data and its interpretation.

Rub (clash points)

Clashes between the partners often came from their background, training and life experiences. These became a valued and valuable part of the research process, leading to more discussion and debate than would otherwise have happened. Language was identified as a key exemplar of power 'rub': while community participants initially felt depowered by academic language, academics equally experienced recovery language as a barrier. Over time, the process became one more of shared understanding rather than merely translation and terminology:

> I used to switch off when they started talking about data this and data that but I noticed now that it was my stuff – I knew what it meant but thought it was all 'poncy crap' and better than me. Talking about how we talked about things was what made the difference (for us all) […] we all learned new words and stuff. (Community partner, lived experience)

Other clash points proved more difficult to work through. Ethical oversight provides an example of an imbalance that ultimately confers power on the academic partner. Academia is charged with responsibility for participants of research via ethical oversight. This inevitably puts the academic partner into a paternalistic role as they are held institutionally responsible for the safety of partners and involved others. Having to impose ethical procedures on participants emphasises the 'them and us' relationship but, at the same time, training community partners to become researchers and comply with research processes felt less like empowering participants and more like making them more like 'us':

It's not that there's nothing to learn but the most important thing that I bring is my experience and that, when I share it and use it, it's good for the research. I (sort of) get the thing about being anonymous but sometimes I thought it was over the top – I didn't need to be protected, it was about visible recovery. (Community partner, lived experience)

What have we learned?

Our work was designed to offer insights and open up areas of investigation in relation to coproduction in research. The intention has not been to reduce the notion of coproduction to a definitive set of variables. It has been to reflect upon and explore the emerging factors which then formed the R Factor Framework; this evolved over time. Our work opens up fundamental questions about the very nature of research, the relational essence of coproduction and its practical applications for individuals, organisations, and systems.

The R Factor Framework contents are not exhaustive but are ones that occurred across a range of contexts or were considered to have a significant impact by the project crew. Our intention is not to describe 'good' and 'bad' approaches to coproduction but to reflect on the experiences of this, and in a manner that models coproduction itself.

Coproduction research has been described as a meta-methodology or overarching approach to research (N8/ESRC, 2016), and could be described as a paradigm shift from a conventional and narrow approach to evidence gathering to a more holistic and broad activity that integrates identification of need, evidence production and application. These reflections on the experience of coproduced research throughout the Recovery Voice in Action project appear to be shared and have commonalities with other coproduction researchers. N8/ESRC (2016) recommends that universities need to change and challenge their understanding of research to incorporate the wider eco-system of coproduction. This means widening the boundaries around research processes to recognise that coproduction starts with the formation of partnerships, rather than a pre-determined research question.

Without the partnership, research questions become dominated by academic theory rather than by bottom-up, community-driven needs. Universities need to take active steps to develop and encourage community partnering, including financial support and support-in-kind, rather than tokenistic patronage. This broadening of boundaries needs also to extend to greater sensitivity to ethical oversight, recognising the rights of representation and self-determined risk-taking of community partners/participants. While right to representation is part of the Social Research Association's ethical guidelines (Social Research Association, 2003), current practice and over-protectionism favours risk aversion over facilitating representation. University governance frameworks also need to incorporate partnership working in research, including financial and administrative organisation and allowing greater flexibility in decision-making, partnership working and incorporating recognised partners within the university.

Commissioners and funders of research are also recommended by N8/ESRC (2016) to widen their recognition of what constitutes research and evidence generation. Coproduction represents a wider way of knowing (epistemology) that in many ways better meets the needs of policy and practice commissioners. Boyle and colleagues (2010) also identify that coproduction needs change in the systems and structures of public services to enable coproduction to work effectively in changing services. Coproduced research can identify key problems, provide ways of addressing these problems, and establish a receptive bed for the implementation of practice and policy change through its processes of inclusion and ecological validity. It has been found in this reflection that, when funder expectations set the agenda for the research, this can be at odds with the direction coproduced research can take, and what it can produce. Coproduction requires greater consultation between funders and commissioners and the research partners, and needs to incorporate agreed aims, objectives and wider community impacts.

It is helpful that the Research Excellence Framework (REF) in England has widened the measurement of research activity to include 'impact'. The REF is the instrument whereby UK universities receive research funding from the Higher Education Funding Council of England. Therefore, the REF standards dictate university structures to support research. REF 'impact' allows universities to widen the required outcomes for their researchers to include activities with social benefit. However, as the N8/ESRC has identified, parameters of 'impact' need to be wider still to accommodate the evidence that coproduction can generate (see N8/ESRC, 2016, p.36 for their full recommendations).

Developing coproduction in health and social care

In health governance, coproduction is still in its infancy and models of working have yet to become established. This may be due to the multiple ways of working that coproduction affords and the variety in its application. However, there are examples of coproductive research in other fields, such as environmental science, that the health community can learn from. As mentioned above, coproduction has become well established as a method of collaborative working in environmental sciences and has generated models of decentralised environmental co-management (Berkes, 2010), representing successful devolution of powers to local governance. Global health is also adopting coproduction to present health promotion in culturally sensitive formats, acknowledging that local communities are already the experts in delivering health interventions in challenging environments. For example, the World Health Organization's 'Stop TB Strategy' (WHO, 2006) goes a long way towards coproduction in empowering and partnering with remote local communities to tackle tuberculosis. Health governance and academia needs, and is recommended (Durose et al., 2011; N8/ESRC, 2016), to continue to explore coproduction and what it has to offer, especially with under-represented communities such as people in addiction recovery.

Conclusions

Within Recovery Voice in Action, the impetus for the research came from people in recovery; therefore, they set the research agenda. The community partner planted a seed of curiosity for people to explore future notions such as recovery and stigma, working within and as part of the recovery community to identify its own priorities based on its own experiences.

A lot of the focus of current national policy is on self-reliance and self-accountability. This has been extended here into the research world through developing a curiosity in individuals and the recovery community itself to make a positive contribution. Our project has produced important knowledge on how coproduced research can work, what support it needs to make it work effectively, and what the barriers are. The R Factor Framework sums this up in a succinct way and provides a checklist and assurance that this is 'normal' for coproduced research. Eventually, coproduced research will be 'normal': universities will have developed infrastructure and organisational systems to support it; academic researchers will be enabled to practise it, and the idea of research involvement will be not only accepted but expected by the people who will be most impacted by the research outcomes.

References

Arnstein, S. (1969). A ladder of citizen participation. *Journal of the American Institute of Planners, 35*(4), 216–224.

Asaba, E. & Suarez-Balcazar, Y. (2018). Participatory research: A promising approach to promote meaningful engagement. *Scandinavian Journal of Occupational Therapy, 25*(5), 309–312. doi: 10.1080/11038128.2018.1541224

Berkes, F. (2010). Devolution of environment and resources governance: Trends and future. *Environmental Conservation, 37*(4), 489–500. doi:10.1017/S037689291000072X

Best, D. & Laudet, A. (2010). *The potential of recovery capital*. RSA.

Boyle, D., Coote, A., Sherwood, C. & Slay, J. (2010). *Right here, right now: Taking co-production into the mainstream*. NESTA.

Cahn, E. (2001). *No more throwaway people: The co-production imperative*. Essential Books.

Coote, A. (2002). *Claiming the NHS dividend: Unlocking the benefits of NHS spending*. The King's Fund.

Cox, N., Clayson, A. & Webb, L. (2016). A safe place to reflect on the meaning of recovery: A recovery community co-productive approach using multimedia interviewing technology. *Drugs and Alcohol Today, 16*(1), 4–15.

Durose, C., Beebeejaun, Y., Rees, J., Richardson, J. & Richardson, E. (2011). *Towards co-production in research with communities*. Connected Communities.

EMCDDA (2003). *Annual report on the state of the drugs problem in the European Union and Norway*. European Monitoring Centre for Drugs and Drug Addiction.

Glynos, J. & Speed, E. (2012). Varieties of co-production in public services: time banks in a UK health policy context. *Critical Policy Studies, 6*(4), 402–433. doi: 10.1080/19460171/2012.730760

Goodwin, N., Nelson, J. Ackerman, F. & Weisskopf, T. (2003). *Microeconomics in context*. Houghton Mifflin.

Gossop, M. (2006). *Treating drug misuse problems: Evidence of effectiveness*. National Treatment Agency for Substance Misuse.

Horne, M., Khan, H. & Corrigan, P. (2013). *People-powered health: Health for people, by people and with people*. NESTA.

Needham, C. & Carr, S. (2009). *Co-production: An emerging evidence base for adult social care transformation*. Research briefing 31. Social Care Institute for Excellence.

N8/ESRC. (2016). *Knowledge that matters: Realising the potential of co-production*. N8 Research Partnership/ESRC.

Ostrom, E. & Baugh, W.H. (1973). *Community organization and the provision of police services*. Sage.

Public Health England. (2017). *An evidence review of the outcomes that can be expected of drug misuse treatment in England*. Public Health England.

Shippee, N., Domecq Garces, J., Prutsky Lopez, G., Wang, Z., Elraiyah, T., Nabhan, M., Brito, J., Boehmer, K., Hasan, R., Firwana, B., Erwin, P., Montori, V. & Murad, M. (2013). Patient and service user engagement in research: A systematic review and synthesized framework. *Health Expectations, 18*, 1151–1166.

Social Research Association. (2003). *Ethical guidelines*. Social Research Association.

UK Drug Policy Commission. (2010). *Getting serious about stigma: The problem with stigmatising drug users – An overview*. UK Drug Policy Commission.

Wehrens, R. (2014). Beyond two communities – from research utilization and knowledge translation to co-production? *Public Health, 128*, 545–551.

White, W.L. (2007). Addiction recovery: Its definition and conceptual boundaries. *Journal of Substance Abuse Treatment, 33*(3), 229–241.

World Health Organization (WHO). (2006). *The stop TB strategy*. World Health Organization.

Chapter 8

Coproduction in forensic learning disability settings

Michaela Thomson, Mike Hargreaves[1] and Shaun Peterson[1]

This chapter has been coproduced by a research practitioner (MT) and two individuals who live in and access support from the NHS service referred to here as the trust. The trust is based in the North of England and provides forensic specialist services to approximately 90 people who have a learning disability, in the form of medium- and low-secure ward areas. For the purposes of this chapter, the two co-authors have asked to be referred to as service users and chose the pseudonyms Mike and Shaun.

Mike and Shaun

As service users within the trust, we feel it is important that you know a little bit about how we got here. We were both admitted to the trust directly from mainstream prison following an association with the criminal justice system and detection of our learning disability by the prison services. Before being admitted to the trust, we both had a difficult journey through the education system, which resulted in us attending specialist schools from the age of 10 years approximately. On leaving specialist education, we both struggled to gain meaningful employment, support and friendship networks, which led to deterioration in both our physical and mental health.

Our learning disability diagnoses came in adulthood, but typically a learning disability originates before the age of 18 years and is characterised by varying limitations both in adaptive behaviour and intellectual functioning

---

1. The names of both these authors have been changed to protect their anonymity.

(Schalock et al., 2010). People diagnosed with a learning disability are more likely than the general population to have experienced traumatic life events such as sexual abuse (Sequeira et al., 2003), physical abuse (Focht-New et al., 2008), and adverse life events, including bereavement (Hatton & Emerson, 2004).

Co-authoring this chapter was facilitated by our already effective working relationship built over approximately eight years of knowing and working with Michaela on a range of research-orientated tasks. Over this time, we have shared many ideas and organically formed a way of working together based on the core values of coproduction and meaningful engagement (Boyle & Harris, 2009). That this happened almost accidentally is testament to the mutual respect we have for each other as equal members of a team.

This approach to working in partnership has not always been our experience. We can both recount numerous examples of being rejected and socially excluded from mainstream society, leaving us feeling lonely and isolated. We feel that the rights of people with learning disabilities within society to experience and access normal patterns of everyday life, such as living in our own homes and undertaking meaningful daily activities, is something we have struggled to find and achieve. We have discussed some of the reasons behind this and feel that society, as we understand it, dictates certain norms and expectations about how people should conform and behave, leaving people like us, with a learning disability diagnosis, in an almost impossible situation, as we cannot meet these expectations. This is primarily due to the complexities of our learning disability and lack of societal knowledge and understanding to support us. This led us to formulate a plan of how, going forwards, we were going to work together, based on the principles of coproduction as defined by Boyle & Harris (2009) and the work of Wolfensberger and colleagues (1972).

Wolfensberger wrote of living in a society that, instead of forcing people to conform to societal norms, adapts expectations and environments to fit the person. We believe cultures such as this provide the basis for meaningful coproduction, especially in learning disability and mental health services, where a person's presentation can vary hour by hour.

Method

The motivation behind people with learning disabilities wanting to coproduce is not articulated enough, so we all felt it was important to capture and record our methods for doing so. Our aspiration for this chapter is that it will make a valuable contribution and positive difference by challenging some of the preconceived notions behind current learning disability research, ideology and practice. We hope to do this by highlighting some of the ways coproduction has worked well for us and offer the reader examples of how they can replicate this in similar services. This includes how we can create effective environments and cultures for coproduced work to take place, how we overcame the challenges we faced, and how we can adapt working practices so they facilitate coproduction as the norm. We felt this was important to acknowledge, particularly in the field of learning disability research, as, admittedly, it can be profoundly challenging but also profoundly satisfying.

Our contribution is in three parts. First, we describe coproduction in practice, as illustrated in this chapter. Second, we show how using learning disability-coproduced research as a topic for discussion and focus allowed us to practise what coproduction looks like while learning about the value of engagement in research. And last, we reflect more personally on what works well for us when coproducing, how we feel about research, and what they both mean for people with learning disabilities, using our verbatim quotes.

Alongside our own ideas of coproduction, we wanted to adopt a model for the work we undertook that brought coproduction and research-orientated tasks together to give more clarity, rigour and reliability to what we were trying to achieve. After some deliberation, we decided on an approach called facilitated collaborative action research (Inglis & Cook, 2011), which we felt best matched our aspirations, aims and objectives:

> It enables examination of the understandings of research, whilst acknowledging participants as experts and researchers in their own right. (Inglis & Cook, 2011, p.99)

Facilitated collaborative action research uses a range of activities and information-gathering approaches to form research ideas, questions, observations and findings. We used the principles of this approach to guide the agenda of our weekly meetings, which we opened up to any service users on site who wanted to be involved. In response, our weekly chapter development sessions were attended by an average of six people. In every session, we began by designing our own Easy Read leaflets, using meaningful words and symbols designed by the group that encompassed what the terms 'coproduction' and 'research' meant to us. We then used this same process to list the topics of our weekly sessions, which included:

- the process of coproducing a book chapter
- how I can/want to be involved
- literature searching
- what coproduction means to us
- how we would advise other services wanting to coproduce.

This gave us a sound starting point to work from and build on, and allowed us to 'gel' as a team and get to know each other better. Our Easy Read leaflets were guided by *How to Make Information Accessible*, published by CHANGE (2016).

The Easy Read leaflets ensured that, if someone had missed a session, we could deliver the leaflets to their ward, which allowed them to stay connected and updated with what we had worked on during the session.

This was of particular importance given the stories contributed by the group, which included examples of feeling excluded by the use of complex language/words, strict time constraints in meetings, feeling rushed, being in the presence of people who had not been introduced, being talked over and having to discuss things of a personal and sensitive nature in the presence of people we did not know well.

This is very much the core ethos of coproduction:

> Co–production is a relationship where professionals and citizens share power to design, plan and deliver support together, recognising that both partners have vital contributions to make in order to improve quality of life for people and communities. (New Economics Foundation, 2014, p.7)

By using our chosen approach, we were able to minimise any such occurrences as it 'encourages open dialogue among participants to explore diverse opinions and assumptions. It enables examination of the understandings of research, whilst acknowledging participants as experts and researchers in their own right' (Inglis & Cook, 2011, p.99).

Chapter development process

Our weekly meetings were held on different wards to maximise attendance, as some service users have limited access off the ward areas due to the secure nature of services. We therefore recommend a flexible approach to overcome the initial barrier of access. We worked with the support teams on the wards, contacting them in advance of our visits to ensure they were prepared. We felt this was important because, for people living on the wards, this is their home and we wanted to enhance their living environment in a positive way by our presence, not add any additional stress. We had read in the literature that there is a risk of this being perceived as 'gatekeeping' (McDonald et al., 2016), but for us it was important to have the support of the ward staff working in partnership with us all. We also discussed with the ward staff before our visits any specific service user compatibility issues, which can sometimes be a problem in secure services. Some people may have mental health issues that can bring an element of unpredictability.

The literature review process

The literature review process was a challenge, given the academic nature of what it entails. We discussed this at length and decided as a group that Michaela would take the lead on this task, given her past experience. Michaela had regular conversations with the group during this process to keep all those interested informed. We suggest similar services use the expertise of someone who has done this before and/or is willing to learn how to access and interpret academic literature. We all acknowledged that, without the expertise of someone who understands literature reviews, undertaking it would have been a major challenge for us. This process requires a person with the expertise not only to undertake a literature review but also to translate academic information into an accessible format to ensure maximum inclusion.

This gave us a valuable opportunity to recognise and play to everyone's strengths. By creating a culture where people felt comfortable to be honest about any tasks they found challenging and difficult, we were able to adapt as a team and agree on personal preferences that matched an individual's skill base.

We went about our review using the trust's library and evidence resources to search a variety of databases (e.g. PsycINFO, Medline and Google Scholar), using the following terms: 'coproduction', 'inclusion', 'engagement', 'collaboration', paired with 'disability', 'intellectual disability', 'developmental disability', 'learning difficulty', 'learning disability', 'cognitive disability', 'mental health', or 'service user' paired with 'participatory research', 'participatory action research', 'action research', 'collaborative research', 'emancipatory research' or 'inclusive research'.

Literature review

We found very little literature relating to coproduction in learning disability research and even less relating to forensic (secure) learning disability services. Although there were papers referencing the involvement of people with learning disabilities, we were interested in papers that went beyond involving people to coproducing with them. There was a lack of detail concerning practical ways coproduced research tasks can be facilitated, including research data gathering, analysing and/or presenting. The literature suggested this is largely due to the ethical challenges posed when involving people with learning disabilities in such a manner, along with the logistic issues of access and effective communication (Frankena et al., 2017).

Issues around capacity, consent and risk were all described as barriers, along with lack of researcher experience, difficulty accessing secure services and lack of expertise relating to this cohort (Conder et al., 2011; Garcia-Iriarte et al., 2009; Hutchinson & Lovell, 2013; Stack & McDonald, 2014). This was despite the numerous important social and scientific benefits highlighted from including people in research processes, such as opportunities for making socially valued contributions and the reduction of persistent health, economic and social disparities (Abell et al., 2007; Gilbert, 2014; Johnson, 2009).

The National Research Strategy produced by the Department of Health's Learning Difficulties Research Team (2006) emphasises the importance of engaging people with learning difficulties in research, not least for their expert-by-experience knowledge but also because of the well-publicised concerns about learning disability healthcare provision. People's negative experiences of accessing healthcare have been well documented (Mencap, 2007). The need for specific guidelines and strategies to overcome some of the healthcare provision shortfalls and promote meaningful engagement in healthcare research was raised by Northway (2010):

> It is also important to remember that, if we are to include people with learning disabilities in general healthcare, then we also need to develop strategies to promote their inclusion in general healthcare research, thus ensuring that their views and experiences shape the development of more appropriate services. (p.364)

We felt this did not go far enough, as papers were mainly concerned with 'involving' people with learning disabilities in research rather than coproducing research with them. And although the principles behind such involvement had good intentions, this was not coproduction. We did find some evidence relating to the role of non-disabled researchers facilitating inclusive research with people who have a learning disability (Walmsley, 2005), and the need for transparency and awareness to overcome the challenges of working in an inclusive way (Chappell, 2000). When these were overcome, the benefits of such an approach to both research processes and outcomes were very similar to those of our working group: feeling listened to, valued, respected and involved (Inglis & Cook, 2011; Walmsley, 2005).

This still did not go far enough, and it became evident that further published work was needed. There remained an evident lack of inclusion of people with learning disabilities in policymaking research, which was due to a lack of researcher skills in engaging people and the research language used.

This highlighted the need for change in research-orientated language that a coproduced approach facilitates. In line with Walmsley (2005), we reassigned the labels 'the researcher' and 'the researched' to 'co-researchers' and 'experts by experience'. This reassignment of titles and language overcomes the main criticisms of 'traditional' disability research that the research is not representative of these people's experiences, as the vast majority of research is conducted by non-disabled researchers.

Although we found literature that stated the need for a change in attitudes and language used, we found little evidence of how this was done. Despite this, there was evidence to support the notion that coproduction in research promotes emancipation (seeking positive societal change) and empowerment (seeking positive individual change through participation) (Walmsley, 2005).

Our conclusions from the review informed what we wanted to include in our chapter and how we wanted to present it. We wanted to fill the gaps in the literature by listing our top tips for both coproducing in general and coproduction of research-specific tasks with people who have a learning disability that could be adapted to other minority groups. We then wanted to capture what coproduction means to us personally, using verbatim quotes from a series of informal focus groups, to emphasise the benefits of this approach and concept.

Our top tips for coproducing

We have compiled a list of 'top tips' for anyone to use who is considering coproducing with people with learning disabilities. We also feel these suggestions can and should be extended to include models of positive support in services for people with learning disabilities, because they make us feel valued.

1. Always assume we have capacity and never underestimate us because of our learning disability. We have all been misrepresented, with the assumption that we either do not have capacity or do not understand what is being said to us. The underlying issue here lies with other people lacking an understanding of learning disabilities and the skills to effectively communicate with us. This is then misrepresented as our capacity issue, which is further exacerbated when our capacity fluctuates, which it can for a lot of us on any given day.

2. To support us with this, people need take the time to get to know us, liaise with our support teams, be flexible in their approach and repeat any information or sessions to accommodate us. During the chapter development, we assumed at the beginning of every session that everyone in attendance had capacity. There were occasions when this would change during a session and/or people would miss sessions due to being unwell, but we accommodated this by producing Easy Read leaflets for distribution if needed, repeating the session if required, and going at a pace so we all could keep up.

3. When presenting information, it is important to use an array of different formats, including Easy Read and visual, audio and oral presentations, and language that does not include jargon or acronyms. This supports us to fully engage with what is being discussed and allows experimentation with multiple methods of communication, which may include role play, technology, including iPads, and flip charts and pictorial references from magazines. We all preferred participant numbers in the working group to be kept low – a maximum of six to eight people was ideal for us. Ultimately, the key to getting this right is to actively engage with us, keep things fun, take regular breaks, provide refreshments and let us lead on the timescales. These strategies not only supported us to engage but made us feel valued and relevant.

4. Being supported and involved in a coproduced way makes us feel we are being listened to. We would like to see support strategies and associated service cultures adopt a coproduced model of care as standard. That this was a stand-alone project illustrated to us that this approach can and should be part of the daily support within the service.

5. We explored different ways to undertake research, the many ways we can be involved and what we can expect from being part of this process. For example, if we have been involved in offering ideas for a research project, we expect some of our ideas to be included in the research protocol, so that our inclusion is not just a 'box-ticking' exercise. We also expect to be informed of any findings if we have been participants in a research study, and to be invited to comment on them.

6. People looking to create a coproduced culture or undertake a specific piece of work based on these principles must from the outset be open to change, accept diversity and embrace evolution. Coproduction for us went beyond research discussions and chapter development sessions to a model of support that we want to be adopted as the norm throughout the trust. In its simplest form, coproduction should be a natural and evolving process that should not be an 'add on' or done in a one-off session, but a way of working with us as standard. It is based on mutual respect and equality of input, and should, therefore, be a valuable example of how we should be engaged with all the time.

What coproduction means to us

We felt it was important to capture some first-hand narratives from people who had attended our sessions to grasp their experiences of being involved in this process. We did this by holding a number of informal focus groups and asking people to reflect on the process in its entirety, with a particular emphasis on what they would recommend to others looking to carry out a similar process.

Not all but most of us needed support to understand what coproduction was and what it means in a practical sense. By discussing ways in which this can be done within research gave us a focal point and helped us understand the concept more clearly. Having this explained to us was a good starting point, but we really grasped what coproduction was by learning together, using research-orientated tasks as examples. These included the role of a research consultation group and its benefits for research projects; choosing research methodologies that meet the needs of potential participants; designing Easy Read information and consent forms, and so on. The sessions gave us a valuable insight into how we can engage in a range of research tasks, create cultures that become the norm and have opportunities not only to be involved or included but also to be equal members of a team.

It felt good to be acknowledged and credited for our work, although not all of us wanted to be named in this chapter. We were able to protect our names but still share our opinions about what coproduction meant to us.

- 'I didn't realise I could understand what research and coproduction is, but I do now. I feel proud of myself.'
- 'I get what research is. It's not that difficult to understand it now.'
- 'I have learnt new skills, like team working and learning to speak up and listen.'
- 'I have really enjoyed meeting up and being listened to.'
- 'I am a researcher. I cannot believe it!'
- 'I'm proud of myself.'
- 'I made new friends.'
- 'I had something to tell everyone on my ward when I got back – what I had been doing.'
- 'I felt at the centre. It was great.'
- 'We are going to use some of things we did on our ward because they made us feel listened to and important.'
- 'I want to keep doing things like this. Thank you.'
- 'Research about us is really important but only if you ask us about it first.'
- 'How does anyone know what research really matters if they haven't asked us first?'

As a group, we feel we have shown the value of engaging people with learning disabilities in both research and reflective writing and that, with initial and continued support, people of all abilities are able to meaningfully engage at some level. The process of co-authoring this chapter allowed us to benefit from opportunities seldom available to us, which include intellectual stimulation, being praised and credited for our contributions, intensive meaningful engagement, increased self-esteem and purpose, new skills development and enhanced relationships with peers as a result of working together.

Conclusions

What we set out to do with this chapter was to use the topic of research and all it entails as a way of 'practising' coproduction. This gave us a reference point and a process to follow and practise. At the beginning it was difficult, as we were learning two different things simultaneously: what research is and involves, and what coproduction looks like and means to us. That some of us already knew about research, due to having already worked with the trust researcher, helped.

From a research perspective, we have learned that we can be equal partners with any researchers willing to adopt a coproduced model of engagement. We were able to practise this and learn the skills relating to all elements of the research process, including development (setting the research agenda and design), implementation (data collection and analysis) and dissemination (control over use and outcomes of data).

By adopting a coproduced research culture, we can create opportunities for all to learn, create equal partnerships and produce shared outcomes.

Coproduction in action increased our feelings of empowerment, confidence, pride, knowledge and awareness of our own capabilities and value. We also felt able to offer ideas, and felt free to learn and grow as individuals as a result – something we believe we should all have the opportunity to do, regardless of how we present to mainstream society.

References

Abell, S., Ashmore, J., Beart, S., Brownley, P., Butcher, A., Clarke, Z., Combes, H., Francis, E., Hayes, S., Hemmingham, I., Hicks, K., Ibraham, A., Kenyon, E., Lee, D., McClimens, A., Collins, M., Newton, J. & Wilson, D. (2007). Including everyone in research: The Burton Street Research Group. *British Journal of Learning Disabilities, 35*, 121–124.

Boyle, D. & Harris, M. (2009). *The challenge of co-production*. New Economics Foundation.

CHANGE. (2016). *How to make information accessible: A guide to producing easy read documents.* www.changepeople.org/getmedia/923a6399-c13f-418c-bb29-051413f7e3a3/How-to-make-info-accessible-guide-2016-Final

Chappell, A.L. (2000). Emergence of participatory methodology in learning difficulty research: Understanding the context. *British Journal of Learning Disabilities, 28*, 38–43.

Conder, J., Milner, P. & Mirfin-Veitch, B. (2011). Reflections on a participatory project: The rewards and challenges for the lead researchers. *Journal of Intellectual & Developmental Disability, 36*, 39–48.

Department of Health Learning Difficulties Research Team. (2006). *Let me in, I'm a researcher! Getting involved in research*. Social Care Institute for Excellence.

Focht-New, G., Clements, P.T., Barol, B., Faulkner, M.J. & Service, K.P. (2008). Persons with developmental disabilities exposed to interpersonal violence and crime: Strategies and guidance for assessment. *Perspectives in Psychiatric Care, 44*, 3–13.

Frankena, T.K., Naaldenberg, J., Cardol, M., Meijering, J.V., Leusink, G. & van Schrojenstein Lantman-de Valk, H.M.J. (2017). Exploring academics' views on designs, methods, characteristics and outcomes of inclusive health research with people with intellectual disabilities: A modified Delphi study. *BMJ Open, 6*(8). https://dx.doi.org/10.1136/bmjopen-2016-011861

Garcia-Iriarte, E., Kramer, J.C., Kramer, J.M. & Hammel, J. (2009). 'Who did what?': A participatory action research project to increase group capacity for advocacy. *Journal of Applied Research in Intellectual Disabilities, 22*, 10–22.

Gilbert, T. (2014). Involving people with learning disabilities in research: Issues and possibilities. *Health and Social Care in the Community, 12*, 298–308.

Hatton, C. & Emerson, E. (2004). The relationship between life events and psychopathology amongst children with intellectual disabilities. *Journal of Applied Research in Intellectual Disabilities, 17*, 109–117.

Hutchinson, A. & Lovell, A. (2013). Participatory action research: Moving beyond the mental health 'service user' identity. *Journal of Psychiatric and Mental Health Nursing, 20*, 641–649.

Inglis, P. & Cook, T. (2011). Ten top tips for effectively involving people with a learning disability in research. *Journal of Learning Disabilities and Offending Behaviour, 2*, 98–104.

Johnson, K. (2009). No longer researching about us without us: A researcher's reflection on rights and inclusive research in Ireland. *British Journal of Learning Disabilities, 37*, 250–256.

McDonald, K.E., Conroy, N.E., Kim, C.I., LoBraico, E.J., Prather, E.M. & Olick, R.S. (2016). Is safety in the eye of the beholder? Safeguards in research with adults with intellectual disability. *Journal of Empirical Research on Human Research Ethics, 11*, 424–438.

Mencap. (2007). *Death by indifference*. Mencap.

New Economics Foundation (NEF). (2014). *Commissioning for outcomes and co-production: A practical guide for local authorities*. New Economics Foundation. https://neweconomics.org/uploads/files/974bfd0fd635a9ffcd_j2m6b04bs.pdf

Northway, R. (2010). Review: Equality and access to general healthcare for people with learning disabilities: Reality or rhetoric? *Journal of Research in Nursing, 15*, 363–364.

Schalock, R.L., Borthwick-Duffy, S.A., Bradley, V.J., Buntinx, W.H.E., Coulter, D.L., Craig, E.M., Gomez, S.C., Lachapelle, Y., Luckasson, R., Reeve, A., Shogren, K.A., Snell, M.E., Spreat, S., Tassé, M.J., Thompson, J.R., Verdugo-Alonso, M.A., Wehmeyer, M.L. & Yeager, M.H. (2010). *Intellectual disability: Definition, classification, and systems of supports* (11th ed.). American Association on Intellectual and Developmental Disabilities.

Sequeira, H., Howlin, P. & Hollins, S. (2003). Psychological disturbance associated with sexual abuse in people with learning disabilities: Case-control study. *British Journal of Psychiatry, 183*, 451–456.

Stack, E. & McDonald, K.E. (2014). Action research. *Journal of Policy and Practice in Intellectual Disabilities, 11*, 83–91.

Walmsley, J. (2005). Research and emancipation: Prospects and problems. In G. Grant, P. Goward, M. Richardson & P. Ramcharan (Eds.), *Learning disability: A life cycle approach to valuing people* (pp.724–743). Open University Press.

Wolfensberger, W.P., Nirje, B., Olshansky, S., Perske, R. & Roos, P. (1972). *The principle of normalization in human services.* National Institute on Mental Retardation. https://digitalcommons.unmc.edu/wolf_books/1

Chapter 9

Breaking down the barriers to coproduction[1]

Kate Pieroudis

This chapter focuses on breaking down the barriers to coproduction. It is based on my experiences at the Social Care Institute for Excellence (SCIE) and more than 13 years of working for a range of disability organisations.

Many things can stop meaningful coproduction from happening or being sustainable (Pieroudis et al., 2019). Even defining coproduction can itself be a barrier. At SCIE, we see coproduction as people who use services and carers working in equal partnership with professionals to design, deliver and evaluate services. Or, more simply, people with experience of services working with professionals towards shared goals. It is a way of working that means power is shared with people who often do not get their voices heard so they get a genuine chance at having a say. There isn't one set way of doing coproduction; it depends on the nature of the project, the context and who is involved, but it can be a useful start to think of coproduction more like a set of values or 'ingredients', as I explain below. If it's working well, it's challenging, but new and sometimes completely unexpected perspectives emerge. This change and the learning are part of the process.

SCIE is an improvement agency. We take research and evidence about what is working well and what's new and share it to create better social and healthcare services. We support people who plan, commission, deliver and use services to put that knowledge into practice. Coproduction runs through

---

1. This chapter is based on a report first published online during Coproduction Week 2019 (Pieroudis et al., 2019). With thanks to Michael Turner for his contributions.

everything we do. We have a coproduction network and a steering group made up of people who use services and carers, who guide our work.

Learning about equal partnerships

I joined SCIE in August 2018 and have since had countless conversations with a wide range of social care, health and voluntary organisations about the barriers to meaningful coproduction. My history with coproduction goes back a lot further than this – I was coproducing from 2006, before I had even heard the word coproduction. One of my first jobs was Consultation Officer with Action Disability Kensington & Chelsea (ADKC) – a small, progressive, user-led disability organisation. This was my first encounter with disabled people who were running an organisation. We were frequently commissioned to run 'consultation' events with local disabled people, usually because the local authority, battered by poorly attended engagement events, wanted to hear from them as part of updating or creating disability-related policy or strategy. I understood instinctively that the people best placed to comment on poor services – who could tell us what a good service looks and feels like and how local needs could best be met – were the people using those services. Rather than passive recipients, these people could be part of the solution, shaping, running and creating better services that actually met their needs.

Over time, I became concerned about the one-sided ask: 'Tell us what you think.' Involvement usually stopped there. There was rarely any feedback on which views would be taken forward and why, and no plans for future engagement. I became concerned that people's views and experiences were not considered valid learning. People were not being properly rewarded for participating and there was no genuine sharing of power, as the professionals retained the overall say on final policies. I began looking for other ways that disabled people's contributions could make a meaningful impact.

Alternatives that actually empowered people included designing 'Know Your Rights' and 'Get on Board' training to support people to understand local decision-making processes and participate in them effectively; joining steering groups tasked with creating disability and equality policies, or scrutiny panels looking in detail at how services were performing, and training people to sit on staff recruitment panels – for example, for social workers – and have a say in the workforce of the future, while themselves developing new skills.

The foundation of such training was confidence building. While some people who use services and their carers had found their voice through previous experience of coproduction, many had not. Some were consistently disempowered by not having their basic needs met, which eroded their ability to believe they had anything valuable to contribute. It fostered a deep mistrust of the systems that had failed them. I built up people's knowledge about how services work, harnessing views so they could be shared in a supportive, peer-led, accessible environment. Some people flourished as their skills and confidence improved.

This reaches far beyond simple involvement and emphasises the difference between consultation and coproduction. Much of my work centres on how best to support organisations to understand this distinction. Language is important as it sets the tone for equality, but it shouldn't be the ultimate focus. Fear of getting things wrong can stop people taking a first step. Action is more important. What are we doing that enables people to have a voice? What values and motivations are driving our actions?

The purpose of this whistle-stop tour of my journey through coproduction and the barriers I have experienced as a professional (who has since become a person who uses mental health services) is that my experiences echo the barriers to coproduction highlighted below by people who use services, carers and other frontline coproduction staff. I revisit these experiences throughout this chapter, supplementing them with research and additional stories, before suggesting solutions and posing questions about the future of coproduction – what needs to happen next?

SCIE's commitment to coproduction

Coproduction runs through all aspects of SCIE's work and is one of SCIE's values. With this in mind, I developed the new advanced coproduction training, using an action learning approach. Action learning is not new, but it was adapted to allow participants to bring real examples of their coproduction work to a session, learn from each other by asking carefully guided questions, and share diverse experiences of coproduction, including barriers experienced and how these were overcome, thereby coproducing solutions and arriving at new perspectives. I hope that, by my sharing this practical method and other reflections as a trainer, others will be inspired to try new ways of working, become more reflective and find new ways to share the power of ideas and learn empathy towards other people's experiences, all of which are vital ingredients for coproduction to happen.

'Breaking down the barriers'

The theme of SCIE's Third Annual Coproduction Week in 2018 was 'Breaking Down the Barriers to Coproduction'. Activities included a Coproduction Festival[2] attended by 110 people – nearly half were people who use services

---

2. A film of the key highlights of SCIE'S Coproduction Festival 2018 can be watched at www.youtube.com/watch?v=qgDxLYegKR0

and carers; the rest were professionals. Many were from SCIE's Coproduction Network, a group of 76 individuals representing service-user and carer-led organisations, individuals who use services, carers and staff from equality, LGBTQI, young people's and other organisations.

The Festival hosted six workshops for attendees. This chapter summarises the discussions and learning from these workshops (and other panel discussions). All of the solutions below are based on participants' views and their insights form much of this chapter's content. Other activities of Coproduction Week included two SCIE webinars that ran web polls on 350 people's experiences of coproduction in their local communities.

Many of the identified barriers are linked, so action needs to consider and address a range of the solutions and approaches to successfully develop and improve coproduction. Eight barriers and potential solutions are outlined. As you read them, do keep this participant's reflection in mind:

> Co-production isn't always a 'natural' or easy way to work. We should see co-production as a long-term goal achieved by having a shared vision and strong leadership. (Person who uses services, SCIE Co-Production Festival, 2018)

1. Lack of clear policies and legislation on coproduction

Most recent health and social care legislation and policy recognises the need to involve people who use services and carers, but there is no legal requirement for organisations to coproduce. There is an 'ethical' argument for coproduction, a basic duty to hear people's voices (see Chapter 12). This compares with the ethical processes and permissions expected of researchers before carrying out a piece of research. Festival participants felt that, if there were an ethical imperative to involve people who use services in the design and delivery of research, this would shift researchers' minds to look for new and innovative ways of coproducing. It might also create space for a legal requirement to emerge from this ethical imperative. There has been recent growing interest in collaborative approaches to research, including a case for research led solely by users (most notably Sweeney et al., 2009). Despite such advances, effectively coproduced research and purely user-led research projects remain in the minority, compared with well-funded, institutional research programmes. Better coproduced research would provide people who use services and carers with more defined roles in developing research questions, such as being supported and trained to become peer researchers to carry out data collection, analysis and evaluation.

I spoke to Niccola Hutchinson-Pascal, Head of Co-Production Collective at University College London (UCL) – one of the very few, if not the only coproduced coproduction centres – about how ethical review processes are not fit for purpose when it comes to coproduced research. She said:

> Co-Production Collective believes that the ethical approval process, a key part of research development, is in need of a review when it comes to coproduction. We feel it's important to work with ethics committees to ensure that there is an understanding of what genuine (rather than tokenistic) coproduction is and, if necessary, improve their processes and ensure that they have training so that coproduced research is reviewed in a fair and appropriate way.

Participants in the Coproduction Festival proposed three broad solutions:

- There could be a legal requirement for coproduction or stronger drivers that create a push for it to happen.
- Coproduced research standards could be developed, complete with guidelines and templates.
- A national lead for coproduction should be appointed in central or local government.

2. Lack of knowledge and understanding

A lack of knowledge and understanding of coproduction is a major barrier. Many organisations and professionals consider it too difficult to coproduce, often believing coproduction to be expensive and without clear benefit, or failing to fully appreciate knowledge grounded in personal experience (Beresford, 2003).

Coproduction is a different way of working with people who use services and carers. It is distinct from approaches such as consultation and involvement (where often key decisions have already been made before involving people, or key issues never make it onto the agenda). Work sometimes takes place with people who use services that is called coproduction but is not being done in a meaningful way. This can lead to coproduction being viewed as a token gesture or a tick-box exercise, rather than it having an actual impact.

More dangerously, research into the recovery model of mental health and direct payments suggests that progressive ideals can become diluted once they are incorporated into an organisation's practice. As coproduction becomes co-opted into the mainstream or led by an institution, its meaning can alter, and people who use services lose power to effect change and have their voices heard.

Several solutions are proposed:

- Clearly define what coproduction means, with information on the principles or values that guide how to do it. These could be developed by national organisations or a network of people who use services and carers.
- More coproduction training and support for staff from induction, and then as part of their continuing practice and development.
- This training must be coproduced – designed and delivered by people who use services, carers and their organisations.
- Develop networking and contact between professionals working on coproduction.
- Start pilot coproduction projects and spread practice from there.
- Produce evidence to show the benefits of coproduction. Monitor the impact or difference coproduction makes.
- Have coproduction champions or local ambassadors with local expertise who can demonstrate how to do it meaningfully, acknowledging the wealth of experience and skills in communities.
- Recognise the importance of developing relationships between everyone involved, including senior managers, people who use services and carers.
- Involve people who use services in all parts of coproduction, from the beginning of the work through to the end. This includes defining what the 'problems' are to start with, what needs to change, having a role in deciding what gets commissioned, designing and delivering projects and evaluating the difference they make.

3. Attitudes and power-sharing

Some participants felt that attitudes towards power-sharing needed to change, both among professionals and among people who use services. Concerns about professional attitudes included:

- thinking things have to be done the way they have always been done
- a culture of 'gatekeepers' – staff having too much control, particularly in places like residential homes
- being risk averse
- believing that people who use services and carers are not able to take part in coproduction because of factors like age or disability.

Such attitudes have a big impact on organisations' and professionals' ability to share power with people who use services and carers, which is essential to true coproduction. Equally, people who use services and carers can have views and experiences that make it difficult for them to be part of coproduction:

- They think it is too difficult.
- Previous negative experience with social or health services can mean they find it difficult to trust professionals.
- They are sometimes resistant to getting involved as they believe they will get into trouble for saying what they think.

Several solutions are proposed:

- Set up peer support groups so that people with similar experiences can support each other and exchange information and experiences.
- Develop a coproduction charter – a set of values or 'ingredients' that guide coproduction, which everyone signs up to.
- Champion a human rights approach – everyone has a fundamental right to participation and having a voice.
- Set up new mechanisms for change – for example, the London Borough of Hammersmith and Fulham set up a Disabled People's Commission to advise on what was important to disabled people. This helped develop coproduction priorities and areas of work in the council.
- Give staff permission and time to build relationships with the people who use their services and carers.
- Give people who use services and carers leadership roles in coproduction, with appropriate support and training.

Coproduction is about people using services gaining equal power with professionals, recognising that they have assets and expertise and that their contribution is of equal value to that of paid staff. Mental health services present particular hurdles. Peter Beresford points to the challenges facing a mental health system 'that retains significant traces of the history of control, detainment, isolation, segregation, pathologisation and medicalisation of people with mental health problems' (Carr, 2016, p.7), suggesting that deep shifts in organisational culture are necessary. Part of this is recognising that roles need to change so that staff are seen not as experts with all the answers but more as facilitators enabling discussion and change.

Negative attitudes often develop when communication has not been right at the outset and relationships have not been given the time to be properly developed. *The Art of Coproduction: A guerrilla guide* (We Coproduce, 2019) emphasises the importance of time:

> Relationships, trust and understanding take time to build […] organisations that take time to build relationships find these last. Organisations that do not find that these waste time in the long term. Ask: Are we allowing enough time to truly transform relationships? Are these deadlines real? Who controls the timescales? (We Coproduce, 2019, p.2)

Time should be taken for everyone to agree on what needs to be coproduced and why, and for roles to be agreed. For some, this will be a completely new way of working. Service users, carers and professionals might all need training to understand what coproduction is and how it's different to what has gone before, and to develop shared understanding of what a coproduced piece of work will look like.

> Co-production is a continuous learning process for everyone. Being willing to take risks and make mistakes, reviewing, reflecting and learning from them, and making changes necessary throughout the process is vital for coproduction. (Carr & Patel, 2016, p.11)

4. Organisational culture and staff

Organisations that try to coproduce don't always succeed in making it a fundamental part of their culture. Making coproduction run through everything an organisation does is often referred to as 'embedding', and it requires culture change. Changing culture ensures the principles and values of coproduction run right through all levels of an organisation's work and become 'everyone's business'. In some organisations, coproduction is left to special coproduction or engagement teams rather than all staff acknowledging that it can apply to everyone's roles.

In some organisations where there is positive work on coproduction, this can get lost when the members of staff involved leave the organisation. Sometimes coproduction work takes place in pockets, in isolation, or only at certain levels, and there is no clear plan to make it happen across the whole organisation.

The following solutions are proposed:

- Ensure senior leadership buy-in to make coproduction fundamental to everything an organisation does, even if this is challenging.
- Make coproduction 'the way we do things'; include it in all policies and job descriptions.

- Acknowledge that sometimes senior managers are signed up to coproduction but unable to get middle management to make it a reality. Staff at all levels should sign up and agree to working in a coproduced way.
- Involve people who use services and carers in leadership roles, both in recruiting leaders and encouraging them to apply for these roles.
- Set up a coproduction team to kick-start and guide coproduction across the organisation, with a view to it becoming self-sustaining.

Frontline workers are closest to people who use services but their unique perspectives and solutions are sometimes forgotten when the coproduction focus is on senior management. All staff in an organisation should be trained in coproduction alongside and by people who use services, making each more likely to understand the other's perspectives, including any barriers they face, and creating the opportunity to coproduce solutions.

The National Development Team for inclusion (NDTi) (Carr, 2016) identifies four main challenges facing coproduction in mainstream NHS mental health services. These are institutional:

- resistance to change
- restrictive administrative procedure and professional practice
- avoidance of challenge, confrontation or emotional expression
- the demand to conform by institutional rules and cultural norms.

Some of the solutions above can assist mainstream mental health services to tackle these challenges and progress towards a coproduction approach.

5. Fear of change and the unknown

Some organisations and individuals fear coproduction as something unknown and potentially risky. Coproduction is not a 'natural' or easy way to work for some staff or people who use services because it involves a major change in relationships and means sharing power. This fear can be addressed by giving staff information about where coproduction has worked elsewhere in the organisation. Support and encouragement from colleagues to try working in a different way is important, especially initially.

Edgar Cahn, author of the seminal *No More Throw-away People* (2000), writes: 'Hell-raising is a critical part of the process' (Cahn, 2008, p.4). Radical changes in organisations and new ways of working mean disruption and asking people to step outside their usual 'roles' and prescribed ways of doing things. It can be uncomfortable, but discomfort is often a sign that it is being done 'right'!

Being able to be honest about these tensions and creating space for staff and users of services to feel heard and have honest, open discussions can help. So too can reminding everyone from the start that we all have strengths and assets and that bringing these together makes the project or service stronger. Working in a coproductive way enables a move from dependence to equality and reciprocity – everyone puts something in, everyone gets something out. For many organisations, this is radical.

6. Insufficient money and resources

As with most areas of social care and public services, there is concern about insufficient funding to support coproduction. Financial pressures require public services to prioritise their work and reduce their capacity to do coproduction. Sometimes decisions need to be taken quickly, or priorities change without allowing time for coproduction.

Often in tough times, organisations are unwilling to try new approaches and instead stick to what they know. Staff who may be stressed or under pressure to deliver targets may lack the ability to take on new ways of working or adapt to them. In addition, funding processes often prevent coproduction.

However, there is a 'bottom-line' argument for coproduction. If coproduction helps get things right first time, it may actually lead to less waste, more efficient use of resources and better services that people want and actually use, resulting in services that are more cost-effective in the long run. If people have a role in shaping services, this may also lead to feelings of improved connectivity to their local community.

There may also be other ways to reward people for taking part that do not involve money. For example, time banking is a system where people donate their time to something and in return receive access to a leisure/social activity in their community – for example, tickets to the cinema or a leisure centre pass.

Solutions might include:

- smarter, more creative use of resources
- make sure there is dedicated time and funding for coproduction
- sharing or pooling resources between organisations to create more resources to make coproduction a reality
- demonstrate how coproduction results in better services over time, with lower costs, when it is done properly.

One Festival participant summed up the potential for coproduction as: 'Innovation is the solution.'

7. Access

Making involvement as accessible as possible is a key principle for coproduction. Yet many people continue to experience barriers that stop them from participating. Access and diversity are two of SCIE's core coproduction values. In coproduction, it is important to work with diverse groups of people and to be proactive about involving under-represented groups – thinking about who is not in the room and why. No one should be excluded from getting involved for reasons of gender, sexuality, age, ethnicity or disability. Crucially, involving people from these groups may provide unique perspectives and facilitate new approaches to problem solving.

The key barriers identified included:

- difficulties getting to meetings and events
- timing of events
- expenses not being covered or paid quickly enough
- lack of access to information or information in accessible formats
- use of inaccessible language and jargon.

People with learning difficulties specifically highlighted problems around inaccessible information and the speed at which many coproduction activities take place, which makes it difficult to understand what is happening and get involved.

Language using technical words and how organisations communicate can be major barriers. It can be useful to create roles for people so they know why they are there. It can also be helpful to embed a shared understanding of coproduction as a group at the start of a piece of work by laying out a shared definition of coproduction and agreed ways of working that show this in practice.

People can be involved with services at many times in their lives, including difficult points, such as when they are ill. People in these situations may need particular support to be involved in coproduction. The following suggestions are proposed:

- Coproduce the format of the meetings and activities so they are accessible to everyone.
- Develop everyone's understanding of different groups of people who use services, carers, different disabilities and long-term health conditions.
- Organise transport for participants.
- Make expenses available on the day of an event, in cash if possible.

- Ask everyone about their access needs in advance.
- Train staff to write Easy Read documents.
- Slow down – allow more time for meetings so that they are not rushed, and ensure plenty of time for discussion. Make sure everyone understands everything and take breaks when needed.
- Be creative in the format and style of meetings and the way questions are asked.
- Work on digital approaches to coproduction, using formats like video-conferencing, but remember this is not accessible for everyone.
- Always make time for the 'quiet voices' and support them to be heard.

Two participant quotes are particularly apt: 'People need to understand it's okay to slow things down'; 'Work differently. Not everything needs "meetings".'

8. Valuing people

People who use services and carers need to feel that the contribution they make through coproduction is valued. People often feel this is not the case and being asked to coproduce without payment can be part of this. People should be paid wherever possible, in the way they prefer. This can help ensure coproduction is a positive experience.

SCIE has a payment policy and helps organisations develop their own. If someone is worried that taking payment for coproduction work may affect their benefits, we offer independent benefits support from Citizen's Advice.[3]

Barriers and solutions in numbers

A total of 364 people attended two SCIE webinars during the 2018 Festival, which explored breaking down the barriers. In the webinars, we asked eight questions about attitudes to coproduction. From these, we picked the six key questions about what the main barriers to coproduction were and what it looks like for people in their local areas.

We had some very illuminating responses (Pieroudis et al., 2019), with the strongest support for legislation to compel organisations to implement coproduction, as follows:

1. 'There is a generally shared definition of coproduction in my organisation or area' – 35% agreed or agreed strongly, 45% disagreed or disagreed strongly and 20% were neutral.

---

3. Guidance on paying people who receive benefits can be found at www.scie.org.uk/co-production/supporting/paying-people-who-receive-benefits

2. 'In my area or organisation, professional attitudes are a major barrier to coproduction' – 36% agreed or agreed strongly, 38% disagreed or disagreed strongly and 26% were neutral.
3. 'There is a good understanding of good practice in coproduction in my organisation or area' – just 21% agreed or agreed strongly while 52% disagreed or disagreed strongly, and 27% were neutral.
4. 'If there was a legal duty to coproduce it would strengthen coproduction in my area or organisation' – 75% agreed or agreed strongly, while just 13% disagreed or disagreed strongly and 12% were neutral.
5. 'In my area or organisation, senior leaders lead coproduction by setting an example' – 44% disagreed or disagreed strongly, while 32% agreed or agreed strongly and 24% were neutral.
6. 'In my area or organisation, people have the skills and knowledge to support coproduction' – 44% disagreed or disagreed strongly, 40% agreed or agreed strongly, and 16% were neutral.

Attitudes and actions on the ground appeared broadly balanced. What would push coproduction forward, participants clearly believed, would be a strong directive from government.

We asked people what would most strengthen coproduction. Participants told us:

- more leadership from senior managers (31%)
- more evidence of what works (27%)
- better funding for user and carer-led groups (24%)
- a new legal duty to coproduce (18%).

Asked what was the most important thing SCIE could do to strengthen coproduction, the suggestions were:

- develop practical guidelines (46%)
- bring together the evidence of what works (29.5%)
- offer more training and support (12%)
- support research and evaluation of coproduction (12%)
- continue to support coproduction week (0.5%).

There are limitations to these findings. Much of the report that formed the basis of this chapter (Pieroudis et al., 2019) was not conducted using scientific methodology; we simply grouped people's workshop responses into themes.

Other limitations include the small number of people who participated, so it would not be appropriate to implement this nationally on the basis of the sample. However, the ideas and questions used in the workshops could form the basis of further coproduced research.

Conclusions

I hope that my experiences and the voices of people who use services and carers have provided practical and imaginative ways to understand and address some of the barriers to coproduction.

Times have changed; rather than asking *why* organisations should coproduce, there has been a shift to asking *how* to coproduce. Rather than adopting one rigid approach that defines values or 'ingredients' for coproduction, coproducing a shared definition and ways of working at the start can prevent future problems. Honesty is important – about what needs to change as well as the limits to what can realistically be changed. Building in time and flexibility, encouraging measured risk – being risk aware rather than risk averse – and supporting staff to try new approaches are key, as these are more likely to generate new, unthought-of perspectives.

Reflecting on my experiences described at the start of the chapter around working with local authorities to better include disabled people in the planning of services, I believe coproduction is all about culture change. It is about equalising the power imbalance between people who use services and professionals, and valuing people's lived experience. It's also about growth and learning – no growth ever came easy and, for many, giving up power is uncomfortable. By having challenging conversations about power, disrupting what's gone before, reflecting on what went well and what didn't and using this learning to make changes along the way, communication and attitudes can shift and ways of working can be transformed so that everyone gains.

The one takeaway I try to impart in any conversation about coproduction is that of the blank sheet of paper. When coproducing a service, project or idea, start with a diverse group and a blank sheet. Ask why the group is there. Explore how the group will decide what should be on the paper. Consider who is not in the room to comment and how to get them there. A blank sheet can terrify some people but, although conversations need to start like this, they do not have to continue the same way. The next step is deciding the format of meetings and clarifying parameters for working as equal partners, where everyone is rewarded for participating. This helps to transform and shift the balance of power to people who use services and carers, as equal partners. It is demanding work that can create long-lasting change and can provide positive growth for all.

References

Beresford, P. (2003). *It's our lives: A short theory of knowledge, distance and experience.* OSP for Citizen Press.

Cahn, E. (2000). *No more throw-away people: The coproduction imperative.* Essential Books.

Cahn, E. (2008). Foreword: A commentary from the United Statres. In New economics Foundation, Co-production: A manifesto for growing the core economy (pp.1-4. New Economics Foundation.

Carr, S., with Coldham, T., Roberts, A., Springham, N., Karlin, L., Nettle, M., Pierri, P. & Watts, R. (2016). *Position paper: Are mainstream mental health services ready to progress transformative co-production?* National Development Team for inclusion. www.ndti.org.uk/resources/useful-tools/coproduction-in-mental-health-toolkit

Carr, S. & Patel, M., with Coldham, T., Roberts, A., Springham, N., Karlin, L., Nettle, M., Pierri, P. & Watts, R. (2016). *Practical guide: Progressing transformative co-production in mental health.* National Development Team for inclusion. www.ndti.org.uk/assets/files/MH_Coproduction_guide.pdf

Pieroudis, K., Turner, M & Fleischmann, P. (2019). *Breaking down the barriers to coproduction.* Social Care Institute for Excellence. www.scie.org.uk/files/co-production/supporting/breaking-down-barriers/breaking-down-barriers-report.pdf

Sweeney, A., Beresford, P., Faulkner, A., Nettle, M. & Rose, D. (2009). *This is survivor research.* PCCS Books.

We Coproduce. (2019). *The art of coproduction: A guerrilla guide.* We Coproduce. www.wecoproduce.com/product-page/the-art-of-coproduction

Barriers and facilitators to coproduction: Conclusion

Mick McKeown and Catherine Mills

This section has challenged traditional concepts such as involvement, engagement and consultation and moved the discussion on to genuine and authentic coproduction. It has explored the multiple barriers in place, such as the issue of consent on the dementia ward, the need to have access to Easy Read materials for people with a learning disability and the issues of organisational culture, resources, policies and attitudes. But it has also tried to demonstrate how barriers can be broken down, albeit with great effort at times. The role of carers must not be underestimated, especially when it comes to care planning when the service user lacks capacity. The need to meet standards such as those outlined in *Triangle of Care* (Carers Trust, 2013) cannot be clearer and staff cooperation is needed for this (Chapter 6). We live in a world where everybody is very busy and has their own targets and priorities. But if this section has demonstrated one thing, it is that coproduction ultimately saves time and resources, and arguably offers better outcomes.

The chapters in this section have introduced some of the facilitating factors for successful coproduction, with genuine human willingness being at the top of the agenda. They have shown that, where professionals have the will, there is a way to achieve positive results. This is no more clearly demonstrated than within those projects that make person-centred relationships real. In addition, attention to prosocial design shows how aspects of place and space might better support human relational care and support. Examples offered from SCIE provide insight into where future facilitators lie, such as the development of policy and legislation that promotes coproduction across all sectors.

Dzur (2019) makes the astute observation that, despite all the powerful impediments, democratic professionals have achieved not-inconsequential gains in enacting coproduction, often in the most unlikely places. He describes a helpful framework for understanding key barriers and enablers. The factors that might conspire to block or dilute effective coproduction include the various bureaucratic, structural, jurisdictional and hierarchical features of public services striving to be effective in simplistic economic terms. Within these constraining environments, professionalism is marked by elite claims to exclusive expertise, the exercise of which remains relationally distant from people seeking help and support. Coproduction offers a means to cut through these constraints and harness expertise born out of experience, inclusively and cooperatively disentangling complex and intractable problems for mutual benefit. In these enabling environments, professional identity is in essence relational, and democratic professionals experience more fulfilling work alongside people seeking help and support. In this way, professionals are agreeably on tap, rather than on top (Repper & Perkins, 2003).

Coproduction is achievable despite many barriers, and we can all play our part in maximising support and facilitation for progressive change. This bodes well for positive, more democratised services, but we must not ignore the powerful inertia to change represented by a homogenous, biomedical psychiatry. Service users and survivors may ally with professionals to enact coproduction or they may prefer not to and continue a unilateral struggle to establish user-led alternatives to mainstream services. This does not necessarily have to be a zero-sum game. There is plenty of scope and need for a plurality of responses, and authentic coproduction within the mainstream must be worth pursuing as at least one of these.

Disinclination on the part of some radical service-user activists to ally themselves to such goals is understandably rooted in adverse previous experiences of mental healthcare and mistrust of the motives and potential of staff claiming progressive ideals. Equally, mainstream professionals will not always recognise themselves in activist criticism or trust their prescriptions for change are realistically achievable. A possible way out of this mutual mistrust is hope in the fact that we are all human and capable of reciprocal relational care and support, and that we can recognise this in each other. Service users and survivors may not always want the help that is offered by services, but in times of crisis they do wish for help. They may, indeed, have been grossly alienated and hurt by previous experience of services. Nevertheless, they may miss contact with services when access is cut off (Rose, 2020). It would be so much better if services were more palatable and consensually engaged with. This is the hope for democratised, coproduced care.

References

Carers Trust. (2013). *Triangle of care: A guide to best practice in mental health care in England* (2nd ed.). Carers Trust.

Dzur, A.W. (2019). *Democracy inside: Participatory innovation in unlikely places.* Oxford University Press.

Repper, J. & Perkins, R. (2003). *Social inclusion and recovery*. Balliere Tindall.

Rose, D. (2020). *The paradox of COVID 19 and 'extreme vulnerability'*. [Online.] NSUN www.nsun.org.uk/the-paradox-of-covid-19-and-extreme-vulnerability

Section 3

Coproducing the future

Coproducing the future: Introduction

Tim Thornton

This final section, 'Coproducing the Future', looks forward to the possible shape of coproduction in mental health services (and beyond) and explores the arguments for it as a goal and how to achieve it.

Inevitably in an edited and coproduced book, the division of individual contributions into sections is an imperfect fit. Thus, issues of exploring and articulating existing attempts at coproduction from Section 1 and barriers and facilitators to it from Section 2 return. Further, in looking to the future, all these chapters in their different ways also look backwards. But this can be justified via the warning, usually attributed to George Santayana: 'Those who cannot learn from history are doomed to repeat it.' However, this is not a weakness but a strength, as looking again at issues from new perspectives promises greater insight.

The chapters here range from attention to existing organisational structures, to moral and ethical values and, finally, to political ideals and the means of working towards them.

Don Bryant's Chapter 10, 'A personal story and thoughts', contains an autobiographical element that sets the scene. Don became active in patient and carer representation to a mental health trust following treatment for depression by a psychiatrist who impressed him greatly by asking, 'What are *we* going to do next?' When chairing a steering group to set up a service user and carer assembly, Don encountered difficulties concerning representation of potential stakeholders and then a lack of commitment to coproduction from the trust. Despite this unhappy experience, Don remains optimistic about the future of coproduction but outlines seven substantial practical lessons for promoting coproduction in the future.

In Chapter 11, 'Challenging co-option', Andrew Passey applies lessons from management science to coproduction. Using a distinction between 'citizen producers' (for example, service users and carers) and 'regular producers' (for example, professional staff involved in public services), Andrew considers whether coproduction necessarily requires the latter to cede power to the former, with the likelihood that they will be resistant to or in some way co-opt the language of coproduction to their own interests. If, however, coproduction is viewed not as a zero-sum but a variable sum, then changing the nature of encounters within mental health services could *generate* value, he argues.

Julian Raffay and Walid Elkharam's Chapter 12, 'The ethics of coproduction', starts by drawing a stark contrast between economic arguments for new initiatives in services, whether healthcare or other, and ethical arguments. They point out that there are many economically successful practices that are clearly wrong, such as slavery, child labour and human trafficking. Similarly, they assert that, however well-intentioned, traditional mental health services are morally wrong and that coproduction is the only ethical way to run them.

In the last chapter in the section, Chapter 13, 'Coproducing democratic relationships', Mick McKeown, Albert Dzur and Pamela Fisher look to the broader political context, both presupposed but also supported by coproduction. They suggest that anything that is coproduced results from democratised social relations and that, where coproduction exists, it strengthens democratic relationships and thus both are a means and a consequence of coproduction done properly. Before setting out resources for thinking about how this might be done, they look to the mixed history of attempts to promote democratic approaches to mental healthcare and broader approaches to promoting democracy, often at local level, and the risks faced. They endorse Peter Sedgwick's claim (1982) that the tools and goals for transforming psychiatry are essentially the same as those required for broader social change and hence the general moral of the importance in healthcare services of the relational over the technical to realise democratic ideals.

It would be against the spirit of this book to suggest an interpretation of, or response to, these four chapters. That is for the reader to think about, reflect on and decide. But to suggest some open-ended questions, with links to the chapters to come, may be of help in guiding that process.

How and what should we learn from individual experiences?

This question lies at the heart of much debate about healthcare, both mental and physical. It is reflected in the resurgence of interest in person-centred care and medicine for the person, perhaps motivated by the rise and rise of evidence-based medicine. Although the idea of a person-centred approach to healthcare dates back a century, influenced in part by psychotherapeutic practice, new journals and book series are springing up, again influenced by a worry that the individual often goes missing in diagnostic medical categories. But while the 'logic' of evidence-based medicine is clear – research based on large populations using randomised control trials can avoid some of the forms of bias that attach to smaller-scale studies – the rational sway of an individual case is harder to articulate. And yet the experiences set out in Chapter 10 seem to carry an individual weight of authority of a different sort to the appeal to organisational theories in Chapter 11 and moral thinkers in Chapter 12. Thinking through what weight they should carry is an instance of a general question to ask in coproduction. One answer is suggested in Chapter 13: in some contexts, individual views should be combined and balanced in a suitable form of democratic practice. In other contexts, however, where arriving at general decisions is not the issue, the obvious weight of a particular view is harder to explain.

How should we think of values and value judgements in mental healthcare?

Julian Raffay and Walid Elkharam suggest in Chapter 12 that a difference between service providers and service users reflects a corresponding difference of emphasis on facts versus values and science versus art. This is an instance of a long-standing debate about mental healthcare. Thomas Szasz (1960), for example, based one argument for the non-existence of mental illness on the claim that, unlike physical illness, it is value laden. R.E. Kendell (1975) attempted to defend the claim that there is such a thing as mental illness by denying that it is value-laden. K.W.M. (Bill) Fulford (1989) attempted to adjudicate by arguing that all illness is value-laden and no less real for that, but that the values in mental healthcare are more contested and so more obvious than those in physical healthcare.

Bill Fulford (1998) went on to articulate and defend a particular version of values-based practice – to complement evidence-based medicine – which stressed the diversity of human values and the idea of 'dissensus' on an assumption that values are subjective and hence the right approach is to give all (non-totalitarian) values a hearing. Julian and Walid invoke MacIntyre's (2007) Aristotelian value-laden notion of virtue and flourishing as a goal for coproductive healthcare. Such a view is not subjective. There are, according to Aristotle, objectively good ways for humans to flourish. So are the values that might underpin coproduction objective, in the way that facts, arguably, are? Or are they subjective? And if so, how is disagreement to be managed? Does the analogy with art – in contrast with science – support subjectivity or objectivity of the values underpinning coproduced services?

What is the connection between descriptive and the normative claims about coproduction?

Descriptive claims say how things are or were or will be. Normative claims say how they should or ought to be. The distinction reflects that of facts and values mentioned above. The 17th-century philosopher David Hume (1739) famously denied that one could infer an 'ought' from an 'is'. He argued that, when people seem to do so, it is always so they can secretly smuggle in a hidden claim or premise that was normative from which they can later derive a normative conclusion. But, in practical discussions about how to change mental health services, descriptive claims about what happens, or has happened or could happen in organisations, which are made in different ways in chapters 11, 12 and 13, are surely of the utmost importance? And yet in a collection like this, which makes no secret of its support for and belief in the values and virtues of coproduction, many of the conclusions are normative, in the way that Chapter 12 explicitly argues that coproduction is simply morally correct.

Some philosophers have argued that Hume was wrong to draw a sharp distinction between fact and value. Also, in practice, when we agree on values, facts can often go proxy for them. (In Bill Fulford's example, the statement that an apple is maggoty *states* a fact but, in the context of a supermarket customer services department, *expresses* a widely agreed value.) So how do the descriptive claims and the normative claims – claims about what is and what should be – marry with debates about coproduction? What, in each case, is the nature of the *argument* for coproduction and hence the nature or sense of coproduction argued for, in both factual and value-laden terms?

This last point may seem a little abstract, but I hope that an anecdote will make it clearer. A while ago, I was involved in inviting a speaker to a conference at the University of Central Lancashire, co-hosted by our service user group, Comensus, to talk about coproduction. I judged, wrongly it turned out, that the subject matter would make the speaker a popular final presenter of the day with an audience largely drawn from a critical mental health background (whether servicer users, carers or service providers). The talk was not a success, however, as indicated by the tone of the questions that followed. Later, I rather naively wondered aloud why that had been so, and one of my co-organisers from Comensus tactfully took me aside and explained: 'Don't you see, Tim, they came from the Big Smoke to tell us the good news about coproduction. They were not interested in our views. They did not even *try* to coproduce coproduction!'

If coproduction is a goal, then those who support it have an obligation – on pain of self-contradiction – to make their arguments for it as clear as possible – where based on facts and where based on values, for example – so that everyone can understand, weigh and assess them and put forward their suggestions, amendments or rebuttals. That way, hopefully, as well as mental health services, the very idea of coproduction can be coproduced.

References

Fulford, K.W.M. (1989). *Moral theory and medical practice*. Cambridge University Press.

Fulford, K.W.M. (1998). Dissent and dissensus: The limits of consensus formation in psychiatry. In H.A. ten Have & H.-M. Sass (Eds.), *Consensus formation in healthcare ethics* (pp.175–192). Kluwer Academic.

Hume, D. (1739). *A treatise of human nature*. John Noon.

Kendell, R.E. (1975). *The concept of disease and its implications for psychiatry*. University of Edinburgh.

MacIntyre, A. (2007). *After virtue: A study in moral theory* (3rd ed.). Duckworth.

Sedgwick, P. (1982). *Psycho politics*. Pluto Press.

Szasz, T. (1960). The myth of mental illness. *American Psychologist, 15*, 113–118.

Chapter 10

A personal story and thoughts

Don Bryant

In the early part of 2008, I experienced what was, for me, a life-changing experience, or perhaps a life-defining moment, but I will come to that later. I had been having trouble sleeping and felt tired and lethargic and couldn't concentrate for several months. Although still working, I was finding it increasingly difficult to sustain my earlier levels and gradually found it more and more of a struggle. I did not really know what was wrong with me. When I talked to people at work, I was told, 'Get a grip, man,' or, 'Sort yourself out.' Things finally came to a head when, for no apparent reason, I burst into tears. After being diagnosed with severe depression, I was referred to my local specialist mental health trust.

Here I came across my first example of coproduction, and I must admit to being somewhat surprised and a little taken aback. At the end of a very comprehensive appointment with a consultant psychiatrist (whom I later came to trust, respect and greatly admire), she asked me what were we going to do next? My first reaction was, 'Well you are the expert, you tell me! I just want to get better. If I knew how, I would not be here.' We arrived at a care plan into which I did have a lot of input. In retrospect, I now realise how important that intervention was, as I felt on board with my treatment. I felt part of my own recovery. It broke any barriers that may have existed between me and the psychiatrist, and instead created an extremely strong bond between patient and professional. There was no question of blurring boundaries or arguing about treatments or any issues of respect. I very much felt that we were an equal partnership, both striving to find the best solution possible. This surely is the very essence of coproduction.

As I slowly began to recover from my illness, I felt that I needed a routine and purpose to my life. Something to get me out of bed in the mornings (and, indeed, the afternoons). I had a wonderfully supportive wife, family and friends but, after a lifetime of work, I needed more. I talked to my psychiatrist about this, and she agreed that I was ready to do some voluntary work. She suggested that the mental health trust itself could make use of my skills. I had not really thought of this as an option, as my knowledge was restricted to acute hospitals, League of Friends, WRVS (now the Royal Voluntary Service) and so on. That was when I met another brilliant woman, the trust's director of patient participation, who inspired me to think of service users and carers as a vital and valued resource.

I was soon to realise that my trust was then probably the foremost mental health trust in patient and carer participation. It had patient and carer representation on its three main board committees, a patient and carer forum and quarterly meetings of service users and carers to keep everyone up to date with trust policies and representation in a wide range of other activities. The trust at that time was one of very few to pay their service users and carers (a nominal sum of £10 per hour) for their participation. This was not a salary or considered representative of the work done, but it was a tangible appreciation of the skills and wisdom that patients can bring. It gave the impression that service users and carers were valued. It brought an extra confidence boost to those who, in the outside world, might not have been treated with such respect and consideration. There was also a feeling of equality, and that, instead of tokenism, all of us were being listened to and coproduction was a real goal.

At the time, I was doing more, although I did not claim for most of my activity. I became interested in research and was invited to sit on the trust's research governance committee (which oversaw all research done within the trust). I also undertook training to enable me to assist with reviewing serious incidents, such as injuries or deaths that occurred in the trust's hospitals or in the community. This gave me a great insight into the procedures associated with patient care, trigger points and the hugely unhappy lives that patients often lead. It also taught me how wonderful the staff are and the close bonds that are often created between patients, carers and staff in trying to obtain the best results possible.

Around seven years ago, my great mentor, the director of patient participation, retired and, as often happens, changes were made. Payments to service users and carers were withdrawn, resulting in the loss of several excellent volunteers. Additionally, communication with service users was reduced with the disbanding of the service user forum and quarterly meetings. However, a members' council, a forerunner to the council of governors, was set up, and I was elected as service user representative. Unfortunately, this did not work in the way I had hoped. Instead of being a two-way conversation, I found I was just hearing reports from all sectors of the trust, with very little scope for discussion or suggestions. Eventually, after a couple of years, this was disbanded.

To try to work more closely with the trust, discussions were held with a wide range of service users and carers about a service user and carer assembly. I played a leading role in trying to make this assembly successful and saw it as an ideal vehicle for communication both ways between the trust and service users and carers. I also believed that this could strengthen my own strong beliefs in coproduction, and that this would enhance the running of the trust and patient welfare.

We set up a steering group to produce an agreed format and procedures for this new assembly. I was nominated chair. We presented our combined thoughts and plans to a large audience of service users, carers and staff. Essentially, we had decided on a structure of geographical representation. But it seemed that everyone had their own, seemingly irreconcilable, agendas. This was horrendous! Carers wanted the same number of places as service users; people with specific conditions such as addictions and Asperger syndrome wanted their own representatives, and so on. We would have had to have a committee of 30 people or more!

Eventually, after some compromises, we managed to reach general agreement on a structure and asked for volunteers to be on the committee. Disappointingly, after all the ferocity shown, very few expressed an interest in getting involved. However, we started off promisingly, with guest speakers from the senior management team presenting and taking questions. At the same time, I was elected to the board of the Mental Health Network, the national mental health arm of the NHS Confederation (which represents organisations connected to the NHS). This gave me a national perspective on what was happening in trusts across the country. I was also the service user and carer representative on the trust's quality assurance committee, where patient safety, participation and coproduction were my main concerns. I was joined on this committee by a carer (who later became a friend), who was on the assembly committee. They shared the same goals of coproduction and participation as I did.

As time went on, I was becoming increasingly concerned about the lack of progress the trust was making about many of the improvements we had advocated. The service user and carer committee had been granted the status of a board committee, which meant that we reported directly to the trust's board of directors. We raised a number of issues that were minuted but the discussions about what to do dragged on and on until they seemed to disappear.

I later discovered that the minutes were never sent to the director; only a verbal update was given by a senior member of staff. I suspect that not all our concerns were mentioned and that our opinions became meaningless when we did not know what the directors had actually been told.

We were, however, starting to have an effect on the trust's quality assurance committee after continually raising the importance of participation and coproduction. My friend, who had done sterling work in engaging the Asperger team, wrote an internal paper extolling the need for coproduction and greater participation between staff, service users and carers. This paper was welcomed by the non-executive directors, who asked the trust to produce a report on the issue within three months. At the request of the trust, this deadline was extended by a further year!

By now I was in a difficult position. I had been discharged from my original illness some two and a half years previously. Under the trust's rules, I could only be regarded as a service user for three years after discharge. This meant that I would have to give up my positions within the trust and on the Mental Health Network board. Although I knew the rules and accepted them, I do feel that a lot of knowledge and experience is lost when continued use is not made of experts by experience.

The report into coproduction slowly rumbled on. Meetings were held, to which I was invited, along with various members of staff. We seemed to have endless discussions on procedures. What was interesting was that all the members of staff agreed that there should be coproduction and far greater participation. Unfortunately, those members of staff only attended the first meeting! Why? I do not know. Was it that they did not really believe it? Was it that they did not have time? Was it that they did not think it important enough or that they simply had enough of more procedures?

Anyway, we produced a draft report, which we were told was to be presented at the board meeting prior to our next assembly meeting. By this time, I had stepped down as chair and was replaced, somewhat surprisingly, by the same senior manager who had thought it unnecessary to forward the minutes to the board. I am firmly of the belief that the assembly should have been chaired by a service user or carer. The ensuing assembly meeting was, in my opinion, an absolute disaster:

- First, we were informed five minutes before the meeting that the senior manager would not be present.
- Second, we were told that our paper on coproduction had not been presented to the board.

- Third, one of the members of staff who had spoken at our coproduction meeting, and seemed very much in favour of service user participation, presented a detailed staff training plan that had not been discussed with any service users or carers prior to adoption. Not only that, but I found the talk very patronising – it was about using demographic profiling to plan staffing needs, which was being considered for the first time. It begged the question as to what the trust had been doing for the past 50 years!

There followed a somewhat fractious and unproductive discussion, with a several of us stating that we felt extremely let down by the lack of information or prior knowledge of why, after six months of work and promises, the coproduction paper had not been discussed. Yet again, we were left with the feeling that our opinions and comments counted for nothing.

The next day, though, my friend and I were asked (summoned?) by the senior manager who had not attended the assembly to attend a meeting to explain what had happened. We were told that a member of staff had complained about our attitudes and that several others and a service user had been critical of our actions. I did not feel that we had anything to answer for and was bitterly disappointed that people had allegedly gone behind our backs and not mentioned anything to us at the time or later. I had always thought that I was approachable and that I got on well with the staff present. After further discussion, my friend and I both felt compelled to resign immediately, as we felt we had lost the support of staff and, indeed, service users (although at all times we had acted in what we thought were service user interests). I felt very emotional as I made my decision, having been involved for 10 years and given everything I could in support of service users and carers. Neither of us was asked to reconsider, so I guess you could say we jumped before we were pushed. In retrospect, I think we were boxed into a corner and effectively forced out, which I now appreciate is a classic managerial obstruction tactic.

When people have been promised so much and let down, is it surprising that this resistance comes laden with emotion? Some of this resistance might be construed as angry and aggressive, but there will always be something meaningful in what is being communicated, as long as others care to hear it.

The sadness of all this is that the assembly has never been reconvened. As far as I know, the paper on coproduction has never been discussed. It seems to me that the managers there wanted an illusion of democracy, rather than the real thing. Some of their ineptness provoked a fractious response and, because of this conflict, the assembly was deemed expendable… And so it was dispensed with. While most trusts have moved forwards on patient participation, my trust, unfortunately, went backwards and is now in a position where there is no direct communication with service users and carers and no outlet for discussions to ascertain opinions.

What I have written here may appear to be extremely critical of my trust – it is not meant to be. Rather, it is an attempt to look at lessons learned and questions asked. I have huge regard for my trust and most of the people within it, especially the executive directors, who have always listened to me and appreciated my opinions. I will always stick up for my trust and the excellent progress they have made in most areas of care – notably in their 'No Force First', 'Zero Suicide' and 'Just and Learning Culture' policies, in which they lead the rest of the country.

Would I do the same thing again? Undoubtedly, yes. Would I do things differently? Most certainly, yes!

These are the lessons I have learned:

1. It is hugely difficult to change culture from the outside. In this respect, I am very much suggesting that service users and carers are on the 'outside'. We do not have the power or authority to change anything; even less so do people with lived experience who are no longer considered to be 'service users'.[1] We can try to influence, lobby or become involved, but at the end of the day we are powerless unless the decision-makers back us. This is why all salespeople want to talk to the decision-makers rather than their subordinates, who tend to promise the world, say that they are on your side, and procrastinate. Very few subordinates are prepared to argue your case if those above them either disagree or do not feel it is important. Many appear to be career minded and very loathe to disagree with those above them. I do believe, though, that many staff who are genuine in their commitment to coproduction and increased democratisation as an idea a) struggle to understand how to meaningfully enact it; b) can be (or feel) unsupported within their environment, and c) are subject to powerful undercurrents of loyalty within teams, to do with self-protection, which are a major barrier to letting go of power.

2. It is vital to have a 'champion' – someone with considerable influence or position who will fight for a principle, no matter what. This person must be able to persuade others, by logic, corporate advantages, ethics (see Chapter 12) and morality that patients and staff must come closer together. It is not easy to find such champions but they do exist. Marie Gabriel CBE, who chaired East London NHS Foundation Trust, then Norfolk and Suffolk NHS

---

1. As previously expained, service users who have been discharged by the trust for three years are no longer regarded as service users but simply as members of the public.

Foundation Trust, and, from 2020, the NHS Race and Health Observatory, is one such champion. She has spent a lifetime improving equality and diversity. Under her guidance, East London NHS Foundation Trust had service user and carer involvement in all the strategic plans, from the very beginning to the published final version. This is the true coproduction that I am seeking to achieve.

3. It is important to engage with staff at all levels of the trust and not just those at the very top. There needs to be a multi-pronged approach. It is unrealistic to expect that people at the top of the ladder will wave a magic wand and everyone overnight will be converted. Change must also occur from the bottom up, where smaller teams can adopt coproduction relatively easily and results can be simpler to identify and quantify.

4. Training is so important. We spend vast amounts of money training mental health staff, and rightly so. We teach our leaders and management a whole raft of management skills in order that they may make better decisions, understand complex data and team building, and even learn etiquette and rules for meetings. But how much do we spend on service users and carers? Do we actually train them at all? If we want them to take part in discussions, if we say that their opinions are important, surely we should provide them with skills to properly engage with staff and governance processes? Why do so few service users become involved in the running of trusts? Is it because they feel that they do not have the necessary skills to engage with highly educated and knowledgeable senior managers?

5. We need a strong and vibrant service user and carer group who are eager for change. One of the questions I keep asking myself is whether service users and carers are interested in becoming involved, as it always seems a struggle to persuade people to attend meetings and so forth. Perhaps meetings are somewhat outdated; they are certainly time consuming. Perhaps we need to think about other forms of discussion, particularly early in the process at the point of choosing the core group and seeking opinions from service users and carers. I am not of the generation that grew up with social media, but I think that expansion of this form of communication would greatly help our cause and encourage self-expression, ideas and interest. I know that many people struggle just to get through the day, but when we consider that my own trust has in the region of 40,000 patients on their records, just the involvement of say 50 to 100 should be achievable. The reasons behind the reluctance to become involved would make a fascinating piece of research. Having said this,

there are examples of critically minded service users who have organised themselves externally to services to provide an independent voice. In Liverpool, there was the Mental Health Consortium, and now ReVision. Their very existence reveals the democratic deficiencies within provider organisations that this chapter highlights.

Where now?

So, what now for me? I still have an abiding desire to help improve the quality of life and expectations of service users; for them to have some control over their individual care and equality in terms of deciding what kind of trust they would like providing the services they need and use. As previously explained, I am no longer considered a service user, I have limited opportunities within my own trust, but I am looking outside of this, particularly to the world of research. I believe that research and evaluation offer the perfect start to ingrain the culture of coproduction within mental health services and, indeed, the wider arena of health in general. Having been involved in research, I have now started campaigning for full coproduction with service users, carers, staff and members of the public, particularly those with experience of mental health issues.

So far, I am pleased to say that I have received a lot of support from the likes of the National Institute of Health Research (NIHR), NHS R&D North West, Liverpool John Moores University, the University of Liverpool and others. All of these institutions have been hugely supportive, and we have now been able to set up a terrific group of service users and staff, who have grown together and set up an integrated research group. We call it the 'Side by Side' research group and it is exactly that – coproduction in practice. Most of the service users have had no experience of research planning or methodology, so we got some training and learned. We also have a mentor from a local university who has given us extremely helpful advice. As our first project, we are about to look at the experiences of volunteers within our trust, and we plan then to move onto other, perhaps more specialised projects, but that is up to the group. It may be that we also become involved in service user-led research as we become more proficient and knowledgeable. I also hope that our members will be asked to take part in outside research, on a coproduction basis, of course.

Research is also the forerunner in patient and public involvement. For research projects to be eligible for NIHR funding, there must be public and patient involvement during every stage of the project. This includes both the writing of the bid itself and the processes thereafter. While not yet coproduction, it is certainly working towards that and acknowledging the vital role that patients can play, not only as research subjects and participants but also in helping to formulate the research itself and protecting the rights of the people involved. As well as being a research ambassador and public adviser, I am on the committee of an NIHR-funded group of patients with chronic health issues, who are all research ambassadors. We support each other and campaign for greater patient involvement in all aspects of research. This is very rewarding and has no boundaries between mental and physical health, illustrating the belief that one affects the other and that, by working closer together, we can break down some of the present barriers between the two.

Another outside area in which I am involved is as a member of a local university's service user and carer steering group, looking at coproduction in the areas of teaching allied health and social work students. As so much of these practitioners' work involves patients, it was felt that patients themselves should have more of a say in the running of the courses, curriculum and engagement. It is very reassuring that nurses and social workers of the future will have a grounding in and experience of a culture of coproduction.

I am extremely optimistic about the future of coproduction. Awareness and recognition of coproduction is ever increasing, particularly at an advisory level. I feel that the intellectual arguments regarding coproduction have been won; all that remains is the drive and perhaps courage of people to make the necessary changes happen. I have been told on many occasions that service users cannot become non-executive directors of NHS mental health trusts. If that is so, surely it is misguided and sad, if not discriminatory. A service user or someone with lived experience on the board of a mental health trust would be a great step forward in every respect.

Health and Social Care Northern Ireland (HSCNI), the Northern Ireland organisation responsible for delivering its statutory health and social care services, has published a coproduction guide titled *Connecting and Realising Value through People* (Engage, 2018). The guide has been produced by Engage, part of HSCNI that exists to promote personal and patient involvement. It explains coproduction, why it's important and how to coproduce, including its principles and specific practical guidance for trust board members and executive officers, policymakers, people with lived experience and peer networks, operational managers and team and clinical leads, and local communities. It states clearly that coproduction is 'an enabler of transformational change' that:

> ... places people at the centre of decision making and aims to connect people together in representative networks so that they can meaningfully influence, shape and participate as real partners in the commissioning, planning, delivery and evaluation of services. (Engage, 2018, p.6)

I'm going to quote directly the 'key implementation steps to effective coproduction' in the guide, but I urge you to download the whole booklet. It's free from the Engage pages of the HSCNI website:[2]

> 1. Build relationships between services, staff, local communities and other partners. Commit to embedding coproduction into work programmes until it becomes the way we work.
>
> 2. Seek first to understand by mapping local needs, assets and experiences. Share perspectives and knowledge. Present data about population needs, trends, services and resources in easily understandable formulae.
>
> 3. Develop common purposes together. Agree visionary goals and outcomes. Establish core values and govern shared decision-making by co-design and co-delivery teams.
>
> 4. Deliver solutions together. Identify areas for co-delivery. Strengthen multidisciplinary team integration. Invest in peer services and in partnerships with others build social capital models of delivery.
>
> 5. Invest in the development and strengthening of representative networks. Build the team by recruiting the right combination of people. Take positive action to include unrepresented groups.
>
> 6. Take time to appreciate the evidence of what works and how this can be tailored and blended with lived experience and with local needs, perspectives and goals. Invest in capacity-building training for the team.
>
> 7. Design together – work on innovative solutions which reflect evidence, experience and improves people's outcomes. Use quality improvement and implementation science methodology to test implementation and bring improvements to scale.
>
> 8. Evaluate together – regularly reflect and review progress and impact against agreed goals. Ensure systems have been put in place to reward and recognise people's contribution. Aim to move from 'You said' to 'We did'.
> (Engage, 2018, p.33)

This could have been my former mentor's words. I am convinced that the majority of trusts, like my own, have been treading water on this for years, making token gestures. It would be interesting to discover how readers of this book would rate their own trusts on these implementation steps. If you feel that there has been insufficient movement, then consider doing something about it.

---

2. www.health-ni.gov.uk/sites/default/files/publications/health/HSCB-Co-Production-Guide.pdf

As I have discovered, it may be painful at times, but at the end of the day, it is immensely worthwhile.

References

Engage (2018). *Co-production guide for Northern Ireland: Connecting and realising value through people*. Health and Social Care Northern Ireland. www.health-ni.gov.uk/sites/default/files/publications/health/HSCB-Co-Production-Guide.pdf

Chapter 11

Challenging co-option: From coproduction by organisations to co-creation of value by users

Andrew Passey

There is a growing interest in the potential of coproduction in public services, as seen in a plethora of academic papers and think-tank reports, and across various policy areas and different locations (see, for example, the review by Loeffler and Bovaird (2016)). Much of the debate has tended to emphasise the positive in respect of the benefits claimed for coproduction. Perhaps in consequence, policymakers are increasingly interested in it as a means towards user participation and empowerment in public services, and as a way to make services more effective (higher quality) and more efficient. Coproduction is often linked with concepts such as service user feedback, user participation, patient and public involvement, patient- or user-centred practice, and organisational partnership working in public services (Loeffler & Bovaird, 2016). There is a risk that the meaning of coproduction is hollowed out as it becomes all things to all people. If that happens, then it might lose any potential to be a means to the positive ends with which it is credited. The risk of capture by policymakers and co-option by professionals and organisations seems clear here.

Many of the benefits of coproduction outlined in the literature are those said to accrue to service users, their families and, at times, citizens more widely. These are the 'citizen producers' in Ostrom's influential formulation (Ostrom, 1996). Less visible have been the professional staff who are involved in the design, management and delivery of public services, and who Ostrom called 'regular producers'. For me, that is a worrying absence, given that professional staff are, and will be, key actors in efforts to shift public services towards coproduction. In short, if professionals are not able or willing to change their views and practices, then however much policymakers and senior staff seek to promote coproduction, it will only ever have limited purchase on the frontline. For sure, professional roles and interests are implied in much of the debate about coproduction, but there is less specifically about how staff might view coproduction, how well equipped or not they are to change their professional practice, or how the contexts in which they work might enable or constrain coproduction (Tuurnas, 2015). Further, there is the question of whether and how they might actively seek to 'capture' coproduction to further their professional interests at the expense of citizen producers, in a form of co-option. My proposal is that a richer understanding of coproduction is needed to lessen this risk of co-option.

This chapter explores some of those issues. It begins by refining the notion of coproduction, drawing on recent work that brings in a services management perspective, and sets out some key points about coproduction in mental health services, including evidence about its benefits and potential downsides. Attention then shifts to professionals working in public services. Recent accounts suggest that professionalism is increasingly about 'relating' (Anteby et al., 2016), which means that, in theory, professionalism is becoming more closely aligned with coproduction (Brandsen & Honingh, 2016). There then follows an assessment of the potential of coproduction in mental health services, including how a focus on service users as the (co-)creators of value in public services might support or inhibit richer forms of public service coproduction. The chapter concludes with a brief reflection on the implications of the discussion and makes suggestions for further coproduced research.

What is coproduction and what does it involve?

The analytical framework presented in this chapter reflects developments in the public management field, in which coproduction is a contribution to the creation of value in public services, but ultimately it is service users who create value in their interactions with public services (Osborne, 2018). In foregrounding the user rather than the service organisation, this perspective inverts the way that coproduction has often been seen and challenges professionals to make a shift. The hierarchy between professionals and service users might itself be challenged, therefore, offering a chance to look again at the potential in mental health services for what has been described as 'transformative' coproduction (Carr, 2016).

This chapter uses a specific definition of coproduction as 'the voluntary or involuntary involvement of public service users in the design, management, delivery and/or evaluation of public services' (Osborne et al., 2016, p.640). Coproduction can thus happen in various ways at different stages in the policy cycle. It can be voluntary, such as when service users work alongside professionals to co-design a new service. It can be 'involuntary', such as in frontline service delivery in which coproduction is 'intrinsic' to the interaction between the user and provider of the service. Different actors are involved in coproduction, and each has assets and resources that, if applied together, have potential to contribute to public services. Service users and citizens bring with them assets such as experiential knowledge, social networks, attitudes, values, and aspirations (Loeffler & Bovaird, 2016, p.1008). In coproduction, they are viewed as active participants in public services, and not as passive recipients.

That coproduction is essentially about parties working together, parties possessing assets and resources, and parties having the potential to influence power dynamics raises the question of winners and losers. If we think of coproduction as requiring one party to cede power to another, then a service encounter will become (or remain) a zero sum. Someone has to lose so somebody else can gain. However, if coproduction is underpinned by a 'positive-sum notion of power' (Durose & Richardson, 2015, p.20), it might generate value that is greater than the sum of its constituent parts. A view of coproduction as being about positive-sum power and the positioning of the service user as creator of value brings the potential for transformative coproduction.

The evidence about coproduction and mental health

Mental health services have not been immune to the debate over the merits of coproduction (see, for example, Slay & Stephens, 2013), although it has been argued that very little of it has been led from the frontline, especially by service users (Carr, 2016). The nature of services and the coercive power of the state have led to questions about how far coproduction can extend. For example, it has been claimed that it is not possible to coproduce psychiatric mental health services themselves, but that knowledge about them might be coproduced (Pilgrim, 2018). New knowledge and synergies can be part of that, especially when codesigning policy (Durose & Richardson, 2015), but that still leaves open the question about frontline services. There may be an issue here around the acuity of need, the complexity of issues with which people are presenting to services and the status of service users relative to one another. Others have been more optimistic (Slay & Stephens, 2013), citing evidence that some mental health services are amenable to coproduction. These different perspectives show that coproduction is not simply an end in itself, such as increasing citizen engagement in services, but that it is also a means to achieve particular things, such as improved services (Loeffler & Bovaird, 2016) and social justice (Cahn, 2000).

Impacts and upsides

Evidence about the impact of coproduction in mental health services is limited (Pilgrim, 2018), although common themes have been identified (Carr, 2016; Slay & Stephens, 2013). Positive impacts have been reported at individual and community levels (Slay & Stephens, 2013), which suggests that coproduction has potential to increase the value of services to individuals and provide wider social or 'public value' (Moore, 1995). Slay and Stephens (2013) identify several ways that it might do so. First, they argue that it has been shown to improve 'well-being-related outcomes' among service users, including 'self-esteem, confidence, resilience, improved physical health, skills and knowledge, problem solving, and negotiation and communication skills' (Slay & Stephens, 2013, p.14). Second, they present claims of strong evidence that coproduction can build individual skills and improve individual 'employability'. This might explain the interest of policymakers as they seek to reduce the costs of public welfare. Third, they note that coproduction has been shown to build individual and system-level 'resilience', thereby giving it preventative potential. Fourth, they provide evidence that it can relieve social isolation by helping to link service users back into social networks, which then builds community social capital. Fifth, they point to an argument that coproduction improves services and increases their impact. It can mean a greater variety of providers and increased time resources and can draw on a broader range of expertise and experience within services, including the lived experience of service users. Finally, they cite evidence of financial benefits, although, as they note, few studies have sought to monetise its benefits due to methodological problems. That said, the policy literature has calculated the financial burden of mental ill health and pointed to the potential for coproduction as one means to help reduce it (Mental Health Taskforce, 2016).

Constraints

Mental health services are said to have characteristics with strong potential to constrain coproduction (Carr, 2016; Pilgrim, 2018). The very meaning of 'mental health' within and outside of services is one factor. Presentations of mental health issues are often complex and subject to social stigma stemming from a view that these conditions represent deviance from social norms (Aneshensel et al., 2013). Services themselves have powers of compulsion and detainment, and are highly medicalised (Carr, 2016). These features are said to lead to partial citizenship and limited agency for mental health service users (Pilgrim, 2018). In addition, mental health professionals are themselves subject to top-down constraints from organisations and managers, and quantified performance measures, which are features of new public management reforms in public services (Evetts, 2009). These pressures reflect the current policy context of neoliberal reform in which the notion of recovery, embedded in a biomedical model, in effect becomes a threshold at which the state can withdraw support as no longer needed (Beresford, 2019, p.7).

Professionals and coproduction

As argued above, the focus of interest in coproduction research and policymaking has tended towards service users and citizens. In contrast, there has only been limited specific attention on coproduction's 'professional side' (Tuurnas, 2015), despite the fact that professional practitioners are crucial actors in any efforts to make public services more coproductive. A review of mental health services reported evidence of professionals drawing on the legitimacy conferred by user engagement and involvement to bolster their own position in the organisation or service in which they work (Carr, 2016). The risk here is that:

> ... [a] radical approach becomes co-opted by mainstream services and becomes absorbed into organisational business, thereby losing its transformational coproductive power. (Carr, 2016, p.10)

In effect, coproduction is co-opted by professionals for their own benefit and/or the benefit of the organisations in which they operate. In turn, users are restricted in the degree of agency and power they might be able to exert within these service systems, at all levels of service use. If the underpinnings of coproduction are insufficiently robust within an organisation or service, there is this danger of co-option (Lino et al., 2019). Further, if user expectations of change are raised in the co-design of new services but then not satisfied, they might be disillusioned (Whicher & Crick, 2019). In these cases, value might be destroyed by organisations and institutional actors in what has been termed coproduction's 'dark side' (Bovaird et al., 2019).

Minimising the potential for professional co-option would require tackling issues of professional power, including that stemming from the specialised knowledge that in part underpins the privilege accorded by wider society to certain kinds of work (Evetts, 2009; Freidson, 2001). In coproduction, other types and sources of knowledge (potentially) gain value of equivalence to that of professionals. The point is not to replace one hierarchy with another, but to integrate them. In that vein, recent accounts suggest that knowledge and expertise are now more dispersed and no longer simply concentrated in embodied professionals or services (Eyal, 2013). This means that, in theory at least, professionalism is more closely linked with coproduction (Brandsen

& Honingh, 2016), which potentially opens professional practice to wider sources and types of knowledge that have potential to challenge existing power dynamics and mitigate the risk of co-option.

Exploring value co-creation in mental health service systems

Recent theoretical work in the public management field has sought to shift the focus from coproduction to 'co-creation'. What this involves is a move from a linear model, in which services and organisations are viewed as the creators of value in public services, to a dynamic perspective that foregrounds service users as the creators of value (Osborne, 2018). This is based in an emphasis on interactive services and not on goods production, which is an important distinction, 'for the inherent reason that public services are not directly generating a product' (Pilgrim, 2018, p.274). Pilgrim concluded coproduction is not possible in coercive psychiatric settings, given that they rest on a limited model of citizenship. I take that argument to suggest that, if the language of coproduction is used in such contexts, it is effectively being co-opted by organisations, services and professionals. However, if we look at Pilgrim's review through a different lens, there might be space for a different argument. In noting the lack of a 'product' in psychiatric settings, he claimed instead that mental health services include encounters between professionals and service users that have a focus on limiting distress (Pilgrim, 2018). This suggests that, in these moments, 'service users are co-creators and coproducers of the services they consume' (Hodgkinson et al., 2017, p.1004). We have frontline coproduction because we are talking about services, not products, but the crux is whether and how service encounters might enable service users to create value.

The remainder of this section explores a typology of processes of coproduction that might enable user co-creation (Osborne et al., 2018). The features of each type of coproduction are briefly outlined, and potential examples from the mental health field are presented. These examples are not detailed, but my aim here is to outline the potential of this way of thinking about coproduction. Further work, across a range of contexts and settings, would be necessary to explore this approach more fully. Mental health services are defined here in a broad way to include intervention on issues relating to 'low-level' emotional wellbeing needs, as well as more acute psychiatric services. Examples are predominantly from the preventative end of mental health services. The key premise is that, by focusing on how coproduction relates to user co-creation of value in public services, professionals and service organisations need to re-position themselves as the proposers rather than the generators of value.

Two modes of value co-creation are rooted in coproduction as an involuntary and inalienable part of any service encounter. The first happens at the individual service level when a service user coproduces service outcomes with staff (Osborne et al., 2018, p.22). While it is intrinsic and at times unconscious, this mode of coproduction can be enhanced by the active engagement of the service user. An example is when a young person receiving talking therapy sets their own goals for the intervention. The key issue is how meaningful the service encounter can be for the service user, given that it might be constrained by particular views on outcomes. For example, if outcomes are pre-set, professionals and organisations are explicitly setting limits, and outcomes might have little resonance for the young person. If the service user was instead able to set their own outcomes (in agreement with the professional) that reflect their own experience, social context and the resources they can combine with those offered by the service to realise the outcomes, then they might be more engaged and the service encounter would help to generate value (Osborne et al., 2018).

The second mode of involuntary coproduction occurs at the level of the service system. Here, user experience is co-constructed in the ways that service encounters are integrated into a service user's wider experience (Osborne et al., 2018, p.23). For the service user, the quality of these encounters 'results partly in their personal experience and satisfaction with the service, but also more fundamentally in how the service experience impacts upon their own life at an emotional and personal level' (Osborne, et al., 2016, p.647). A relating mode of professional practice (Anteby et al., 2016) is implicit here. It points to a need to attend to the relational nature of coproduction and value co-creation, given that, along with the material reality of service settings and their physical environment, 'coproduction as it attempts to create public value is constituted by subjective realities, situated within relationships between producers and users' (Williams et al., 2016, p.710). Osborne and colleagues (2018) provide the example of a person with more acute mental health issues, who will bring their own life experience into their encounters with the service system. Their interactions with services will reflect on them and be reflected upon by them, in ways that will shape their own experiences. According to the authors, the service offer needs to resonate with the wider life experience and social context of the service user if they are to engage with it in ways that might make encounters meaningful and generate value.

Two other modes view coproduction as a voluntary activity by service users. The first, at the single-service level, focuses on 'how value is created for service users by their conscious *co–management* of their individual service experience' (Osborne et al., 2018, p.23, original italics). An example might be a service involving children delivering lessons about mental health and wellbeing to their peers in school, either on their own or alongside professionals. The children involved in delivering the lessons would be co-managing the service. Evidence from the Mental Health Foundation suggests that children find peer educators more credible sources of information than adult educators.[1] Children are reported to be more willing and comfortable to ask questions and explore issues with peers, and the educators (co-managers) themselves can improve their own confidence and esteem, which has potential community benefits that extend beyond the classroom. It might help to build social capital. This has potential to challenge existing power dynamics in public services, but how far it creates value 'will be dependent upon the extent to which there is genuine coproduction between service users and staff' (Osborne et al., 2018, p.23). In other words, control needs to be balanced between professionals and children, which might enable children to increase their individual capacity and capability and the collective capacity and capability of their peers.

The second type of voluntary coproduction is at the service system level. Here, service users work with professionals to co-design services or co-innovate new ways of delivering services (Osborne et al, 2018, p.23). An example might be service users setting research objectives and designing research to generate knowledge that meets their own priorities for new mental health services. This may involve professionals applying their specialised knowledge and expertise as 'agents of a patient-dictated research agenda' (Mader et al., 2018, p.6). Users of services would have the necessary power to design the research that would underpin new services in ways that would align with their experiences (and might also be involved as coproducers of the research). In these ways, an ecology of user and professional knowledge would be recognised and used. This kind of coproductive work to design and innovate public services has potential to build resilience in the wider mental health service system by better orientating it towards users of services. Thus, in consequence of the ways that services and ways of service delivery have been coproduced, they would, in theory, better enable users to co-create value as they interact with them and integrate them with their own resources.

Conclusions and implications

In this chapter, I have suggested that recent work on coproduction that has integrated a services management perspective into thinking about the management of public services (Osborne et al., 2018) has potential to shift perspectives on coproduction in public services, potentially including mental

---

1. www.mentalhealth.org.uk/projects/peer-education-project-pep

health services. By foregrounding service users as the (co-)creators of value in public services, this approach asks questions of organisations and professionals alike. It views coproduction as an inherent part of service encounters between service users and staff working in public service systems because the focus here is on services, not products. That does not, however, necessarily reflect the way that professionals have been educated and trained, or the prevailing perspective of the service systems and organisations in which they work. While evidence suggests involving people who use services in educating and training professionals is a means to foster more trust between them (Beresford, 2019), there is still the issue of changing practice once professionals are working in, and potentially constrained by, public-service systems that are subject to neoliberalism and the pressures of new public management (Evetts, 2009).

One starting point might be to ask what professionals now need to work coproductively in the complex systems that characterise today's public policy and public services. At both broad and narrow levels, change seems necessary, given an argument that 'transformative co-production [...] means disrupting traditional fixed roles and power relations between professionals and service users' (Carr, 2016, p.2). Such a disruption might include moving on from privileging specialised and technical skills and competences that are often associated with professional practice. Instead, in coproduction, 'competences required from the professionals are relational, focusing on the ability to facilitate and mobilise others, rather than technical skills or substantive knowledge of the subject at hand' (Steen & Tuurnas, 2018, p.83). The key word here is *relational*.

I would argue, however, that professionals need to possess a combination of specialised and relational skills and competences if they are to coproduce public services with the people who use them. Such skills and competences would become part of a wider ecology of knowledge, skills and competences that would extend beyond professionals. A focus on relational skills would also link with recent understandings from studies of contemporary professionalism as being increasingly about a relating mode of practice (Anteby et al., 2016). This orientation, linked with a perspective that sees the users of services (and not professionals) as the creators of value in public services, opens potential avenues for more transformative coproduction. At the heart of this is the need for coproduction and value co-creation to be legitimated in the professional practice of people working in public service systems. The relational competences highlighted by Steen and Tuurnas (2018) would be emphasised, within something resembling an ecology of knowledge.

The issue of co-option by professionals and organisations still looms, however. While a recognition that coproduction needs relational competences is helpful, whether it manifests in transformative coproduction rests in part on what 'the ability to facilitate and mobilise others' (Steen & Tuurnas, 2018, p.83) means and how it is done. If it entails pushing responsibility onto service users as services are cut, under the guise of coproduction, then facilitation and mobilisation might lead to co-option. Instead, transformative coproduction would seem to require of professionals and managers that they build their own reflexive capacity and their openness to 'critical review of their professional norms, organisational or institutional processes, and past and present policies and practices' (Williams et al., 2016, p.710). A recent review of whether mainstream mental health services were ready for transformative coproduction identified 'facilitated space to meet and open up dialogue outside the system' (Carr, 2016, p.24) as one potential route towards coproduction. Such a dialogue, the author argued, should include service users, as well as survivors and professionals. This suggests that the kind of critical review called for by Williams and colleagues (2016) should not simply be the preserve of professionals and managers.

In summary, I have suggested the potential for a professional ethos that foregrounds users as the creators of value in public services, and a relating mode of professionalism that facilitates and enables service users to do so in processes of coproduction. This will require more coproduced research about what professionalism would mean in that context. As others have suggested, this might include exploring what professionals do to coproduce services, unpicking the complexity of what is involved in co-creation, and examining how individual professions might shape professional motivations to coproduce (Steen & Tuurnas, 2018, p.88). The point is to better understand the capacity and capability of professionals to re-orientate their practice, given that evidence suggests they will need help and guidance if coproduction is to become embedded (Tuurnas, 2015).

This suggests we need to better understand how constraints from professional cultures might be addressed to realise transformative coproduction. It also means that we need to consider what coproduction and co-creation mean to professional staff in specific contexts, to challenge some of the normative assumptions in the policy literature. Finally, there is more to do to better link the idea of professionalism as a relating mode of practice with an orientation that foregrounds service users as the (co-)creators of value in public services. This might involve applying and appraising the approach outlined in this chapter in different mental health services and settings.

References

Aneshensel, C.S., Phelan, J.C. & Bierman, A. (2013). The sociology of mental health: Surveying the field. In C.S. Aneshensel, J.C. Phelan & A. Bierman (Eds.), *Handbook of the sociology of mental health* (pp.1–19). Springer.

Anteby, M., Chan, C.K. & DiBenigno, J. (2016). Three lenses on occupations and professions in organizations: Becoming, doing, and relating. *The Academy of Management Annals, 10*(1), 183–244.

Beresford, P. (2019). Public participation in health and social care: Exploring the co-production of knowledge. *Frontiers in Sociology, 3*, 41. doi: 10.3389/fsoc.2018.00041

Bovaird, T., Flemig, S., Loeffler, E. & Osborne, S.P. (2019). How far have we come with co-production – and what's next? *Public Money and Management, 39*(4), 229–232.

Brandsen, T. & Honingh, M. (2016). Distinguishing different types of coproduction: A conceptual analysis based on the classical definitions. *Public Administration Review, 76*(3), 427–435.

Cahn, E.S. (2000). *No more throw-away people: The co-production imperative.* Essential Books.

Carr, S., with Coldham, T., Roberts, A., Springham, N., Karlin, L., Nettle, M., Pierri, P. & Watts, R. (2016). *Position paper: Are mainstream mental health services ready to progress transformative co-production?* National Development Team for Inclusion: Bath. www.ndti.org.uk/resources/useful-tools/coproduction-in-mental-health-toolkit

Durose, C. & Richardson, L. (2015). *Designing public policy for co-production: Theory, practice and change.* Policy Press.

Evetts, J. (2009). New professionalism and new public management: Changes, continuities and consequences. *Comparative Sociology, 8*(2), 247–266.

Eyal, G. (2013). For a sociology of expertise: The social origins of the autism epidemic. *American Journal of Sociology, 118*(4), 863–907.

Freidson, E. (2001). *Professionalism, the third logic: On the practice of knowledge.* University of Chicago Press.

Hodgkinson, I.R., Hannibal, C., Keating, B.W., Chester Buxton, R. & Bateman, N. (2017). Toward a public service management: Past, present, and future directions. *Journal of Service Management, 28*(5), 998–1023.

Lino, A.F., Busanelli de Aquino, A.C., de Azevedo, R.R. & Brumatti, L.M. (2019). From rules to collaborative practice: When regulatory mechanisms drive collective co-production. *Public Money and Management, 39*(4), 280–289.

Loeffler, E. & Bovaird, T. (2016). User and community co-production of public services: What does the evidence tell us? *International Journal of Public Administration, 39*(13), 1006–1019.

Mader, L.B., Harris, T., Kläger, S., Wilkinson, I.B. & Hiemstra, T.F. (2018). Inverting the patient involvement paradigm: Defining patient led research. *Research Involvement and Engagement, 4*(1), 21. https://doi.org/10.1186/s40900-018-0104-4

Mental Health Taskforce. (2016). *The five year forward view for mental health.* NHS England. www.england.nhs.uk/wp-content/uploads/2016/02/Mental-Health-Taskforce-FYFV-final.pdf

Moore, M.H. (1995). *Creating public value: Strategic management in government.* Harvard University Press.

Osborne, S.P. (2018). From public service-dominant logic to public service logic: Are public service organizations capable of co-production and value co-creation? *Public Management Review, 20*(2), 225–231.

Osborne, S.P., Radnor, Z. & Strokosch, K. (2016). Co-production and the co-creation of value in public services: A suitable case for treatment? *Public Management Review, 18*(5), 639–653.

Osborne, S.P., Strokosch, K. & Radnor, Z. (2018). Co-production and the co-creation of value in public services: A perspective from service management. In T. Brandsen, T. Steen & B. Verschuere (Eds.), *Co-production and co-creation: Engaging citizens in public services* (pp.18–26). Routledge.

Ostrom, E. (1996). Crossing the great divide: Coproduction, synergy, and development. *World Development, 24*(6), 1073–1087.

Pilgrim, D. (2018). Co-production and involuntary psychiatric settings. *Mental Health Review Journal, 23*(4), 269–279.

Slay, J. & Stephens, L. (2013). *Co-production in mental health: A literature review.* New Economics Foundation.

Steen, T. & Tuurnas, S. (2018). The roles of the professional in co-production and co-creation processes. In T. Brandsen, T. Steen & B. Verschuere (Eds.), *Co-production and co-creation: Engaging citizens in public services* (pp.80–92). Routledge.

Tuurnas, S. (2015). Learning to co-produce? The perspective of public service professionals. *International Journal of Public Sector Management, 28*(7), 583–598.

Whicher, A. & Crick, T. (2019). Co-design, evaluation and the Northern Ireland innovation lab. *Public Money and Management, 39*(4), 290–299.

Williams, B.N., Kang, S.-C. & Johnson, J. (2016). (Co)-contamination as the dark side of co-production: Public value failures in co-production processes. *Public Management Review, 18*(5), 692–717.

Chapter 12

The ethics of coproduction: Stumbling across the light

Julian Raffay and Walid Elkharam

Anyone hoping to show that coproduction is value for money faces a difficult task. Slay and Stephens (2013), for instance, merely assume that coproduction is desirable. Very wisely, they sidestep evidencing that coproduced services are cheaper than traditionally delivered ones. Of course, consultation is expensive and time-consuming. Of course, military-style command-and-control systems are quicker. Undoubtedly, the Light Brigade offered value for money and was efficiently despatched, although with devastating consequences (Adkin, 2004).

If we are arguing economics, there are many contemporary ways of making a fast buck that are clearly wrong: slavery, child labour, human trafficking – we could continue. They are all extremely profitable to those willing to exploit others. Thankfully, most people would simply declare them unacceptable. Similarly, we propose that, however well-intentioned they may be, traditionally delivered services are quite simply wrong. Indeed, we hope that, in the years ahead, coproduction will be considered the only ethical way to run mental health services.

Please do not think we are likening nurses, doctors, social workers, occupational therapists, chaplains and others to slave traders. That would be unwarranted and quite destructive. It is not the staff we have an issue with but what the Schizophrenia Commission declared a 'broken and demoralised system' (2012, p.4). We propose that it is 'broken and demoralised' because, in Peplau's (1988) terms, the 'science' has eclipsed the 'art' of nursing, with devastating consequences. A perfect storm has turned 'nurses into technicians and patients into data' (Raffay, 2012a, p.39), leaving many to conclude that 'the most important thing nurses can do is abandon their training' (Forrest et al., 2000). At the organisational level, we see imminent risk of further Mid Staffordshire-type[1] failures (Francis, 2013), and we propose that coproduction offers us the best safeguard from the tyranny of excessive targets.

In this chapter, we show what led us to conclude that we need to hardwire service user and carer perspectives into mental health service evaluation. In doing so, we argue that ethics provide us with our strongest argument for advancing coproduction. We then pick up Moore's (2017) application of MacIntyre's (2007) ideas to organisations. Moore argues that stressing fact to the detriment of value exposes managers and organisations to failure (as in Mid-Staffordshire).[2] Thence, we suggest service user preferences can help organisations by rebalancing fact with value. And finally, we explore Salvador-Carulla, Lukersmith and Sullivan's (2017) paper, which proposes a broader evidence base for clinical decisions.

Contrasting evidence

What we most like about Slay and Stephens' (2013, p.11) definition of coproduction is their assertion that different partners offer 'vital' contributions. We found this strikingly evident in a paper suggesting that staff may have different priorities from service users (Walsh et al., 2013). This latter study found an 80% error in patient records around 'religious and spiritual concerns' (p.153). For us, this invites critical reflection on how we deliver services and our underlying assumptions and warrants exploration in detail.

Walsh and colleagues compared service users' recollections of their interactions with staff around spirituality with staff reports in the electronic patient records. They concluded:

> The majority of Care Coordinators are unable to see the relevance of spiritual or religious concerns, or feel incompetent to record them faithfully. (Walsh et al., 2013, p.161)

They argued that the 80% error rate suggests a neglect of matters important to service users that is likely to have 'a negative impact upon their overall care and well-being' (Walsh et al., 2013, p.162). Most significantly for our purposes, they recognised that a service driven by service user concerns might differ from common practice. They recommended:

> The Care Plan should be regularly reviewed with the service user concerned; and [...] the service user may be encouraged to articulate their

---

1. The trust was closed down, having been found guilty of mismanagement by a public inquiry.
2. MacIntyre's 'fact' and 'value' broadly correspond to Peplau's 'art' and 'science' respectively.

religious and spiritual concerns and practices in their own terms rather than those supplied by the database and/or Care Coordinator. (p.162)

Raffay's (2012b) grounded theory study suggests an explanation for staff inattention to service user concerns. It proposed that too many demands, including 'evidence-based practice, fear of litigation, quality measures, clinical commissioning, and the threat of private competition', prevent staff from being more responsive to service users (p.75). It further argued that 'interest in spiritual care in mental health is, to a large degree, a response to the perfect storm – a call for a more humane approach to care' (p.74).

Partial evidence-based medicine

Corroboratory evidence emerged from another study exploring why people with mental health problems often approach faith communities as their first port of call (Wonders, 2011). Wonders observed:

> [Faith] Minsters don't have tight boundaries, whereas often the NHS is absolutely screaming with boundaries and I think that there are plusses and minuses to both [...] and I think you have a lot of burnt out [faith] Ministers who don't know how to put any boundaries in and I think you have some NHS healthcare professionals that can't do diddly squat because some rule has said they can't and that is a real shame. (p.81)

Wonders described tight knowledge boundaries reinforcing relational boundaries. She suggested 'the scientific domain still holds precedent, and there is some indication that spirituality is at best tolerated or worked with inconsistently or, at worst, avoided or side-lined' (2011, pp.34–35). She implied that valuing religion and spirituality suggests bias, whereas sidelining them is neutral (Wonders, 2011, p.21). Banicki (2014) (though commenting on positive psychology) alerts us to the hazard:

> The scientific ideal of contemporary social science, namely, can be most revealingly read not as an isolated entity, but rather as one emerging from and pervaded by Western culture. Positive psychology overtly and enthusiastically endorses this ideal, so despite its best intentions to become a culture-free, universally applicable, and normatively neutral science, it turns out to be 'pervaded by Western cultural values and assumptions' [...]. This fact, importantly, is usually unacknowledged and remains hidden, not only from the general public view but also from the theoretical self-awareness of positive psychologists. (p.23)

When 'science' alleges neutrality, entire domains important to service users – not just spirituality – risk being omitted from practice. Duncan and colleagues' *The Heart and Soul of Change* provides substantial evidence that service user perspectives are vital (Duncan et al., 2010). Evidence-based medicine is invaluable, provided its evidence base is broad enough.

Centring services on patient agency

The problem with the biopsychosocial model arises from its 'restricted and simplistic approach to scientific knowledge' (Fernandez et al., 2015, p.1). Restricting biomedical ethics to what clinicians do creates distortions. One such distortion is the conventional framing of evidence-based practice. While clinician agency may legitimately be central in emergency medicine, research suggests its insufficiency elsewhere (Forrest et al., 2000; King's Fund, 2011; Raffay et al., 2016; Sullivan, 2017).

Services are likely to be different if, rather than basing practice on the clinician's sole agency, we start from the basis that service users, carers and staff all have agency. Sullivan argues that recognising service user agency improves effectiveness (Sullivan, 2017, p.13). We support his claim 'that patients are trapped inside the descriptions provided by their physicians' (p.66). Our argument, however, explores the ethical and organisational impacts of service user and carer agency (pp.65–70). By robustly asserting mutual responsibility for shaping services and deciding outcomes, we firmly reject antipsychiatry and the tug of war Sullivan condemns (p.78). However, we disagree with Sullivan when he suggests that 'health is best understood as a goal internal to the practice of medicine', for that places clinicians above other legitimate stakeholders (p.105). This represents a dangerous medical invasion of human distress (Barker, 2003; Brennan, 2004, p.500; Sullivan, 2017). Kitwood's seminal work on dementia, subtitled *The Person Comes First*, recognised fact (organic brain decay), yet argued for a value-based approach (Kitwood, 1997). He understood the difference between a broken leg and a broken heart.

This simplistic distinction between a broken leg and a broken heart challenges how mental health services view service users. Faith communities' continuing role suggests people with mental health problems see them as offering something mental health services cannot (or choose not to) see or deliver. Closer examination suggests evidence-based medicine masks interests and may disadvantage service users, especially in chronic conditions. This argument does not depend on the few studies thus mentioned. It fits the broader debate advanced by the influential philosopher MacIntyre (2007). MacIntyre argues that our culture has lost sight of its foundations. We suggest that few clinicians understand the scientific method's strengths and weaknesses. We infer that mental health services and faith communities, highlighting fact and value respectively, speak different languages and have lost the phrasebook.

Conceptual fragmentation

MacIntyre's *After Virtue* (2007) asserts the legitimacy of service user, carer and staff agency over supposedly indisputable utilitarian truth claims (p.64). At this point, we outline MacIntyre's argument to suggest that excessive erring on the side of fact or value by mental health services and faith communities respectively risks failure. MacIntyre proposed that religion's eventual failure to provide a shared language gave way to the Enlightenment's similar failure (pp.50, 60). He proposes confusion occurs because 'almost everyone, philosopher and non-philosopher alike', implies otherwise (p.68).

Without goal or purpose, MacIntyre (2007) argues, fact becomes uncoupled from morality, leaving only the 'incoherent fragments of a once coherent scheme of thought and action' (pp.55). These 'incoherent fragments' are the problem with the science underpinning evidence-based medicine. It is terrain far too disorientating for the 'theoretical self-awareness' of most clinicians (Banicki, 2014, p.23). Aspiring towards value-neutrality and lacking anchors, many scientifically minded people find worth in the measurable and accept utilitarianism uncritically. Regrettably for service users, 'not everything that counts can be measured. Not everything that can be measured counts' (Cameron, 1963, p.13).

MacIntyre (2007) rejects the idea that services should offer the greatest advantage to the greatest number. He suggests the 'polymorphous character of pleasure and happiness' renders utilitarianism 'a pseudo-concept available for a variety of ideological uses' (p.64). By this, he means that, if we cannot tally happiness units, efforts at sharing out goods (not to mention vast armies of managers, accountants, and clerks) become questionable. Tallying happiness units is particularly problematic when we find ourselves squeezed into someone else's framework. A sighted person, for instance, might resent receiving a succession of trained guide dogs. MacIntyre advises that, when others propose utilitarianism, 'it is always necessary to ask what actual project or purpose is being concealed by its use' (p.64).

Why values matter in mental health

MacIntyre sees our society fragmented by 'too many disparate and rival moral concepts' and bound to fail (2007, p.252). He proposes that 'the Aristotelian moral tradition is the best example we possess of a tradition whose adherents are rationally entitled to a high measure of confidence in its epistemological resources' (p.277). Put more simply, he proposes that virtue focused on the community (rather than the individual) offers the only sure footing for an ethical argument.

Virtue as a protective factor in organisations

Here, we draw on Moore (2017) to contend that: a) failure is pervasive and due to organisation, and b) virtue is a protective factor. If mental health service failure were an abstract threat, virtue ethics might be idealistic, yet failure is pervasive (Schizophrenia Commission, 2012, p.3). Moore proposes that virtue rather than technocracy offers organisations the best protection from failure. He cites Hinings and Mauws (2006) who, responding to church and healthcare provider failures, argue:

> The events in question were in fact *made possible* by well-accepted and highly regarded organizational practices. It is because these organizations were as well organized as they were that these events took place [...] The implication of this explanation is that it applies to the phenomenon of 'organization' itself and, thus, potentially *all* organizations. (Moore, 2017, p.24; original italics)

Moore sees organisational hierarchy replacing moral with technical responsibility – namely, 'turning nurses into technicians and patients into data' (Moore, 2017, p.25; Raffay, 2012b, p.74). Hall (2011) pinpoints the specific factors within the virtue tradition that can mitigate this vulnerability:

> More than the comparatively thin or limited notions of utilitarian happiness or the socially contracted justice of reciprocal tolerance, Aristotle and MacIntyre develop the concept of human flourishing (*eudaimonia*) as a thick or full notion of genuine happiness, health, integration, and harmony. (p.124)

Moore argues that virtuous organisations ensure internal goods (compassionate care) take precedence over external goods (targets). His organisational ethics perspective lifts our horizons beyond the clinician–patient pairing, towards the community. He reveals features central to our argument yet invisible to evidence-based medicine's individualistic focus.

Service user preferences as a protective factor

Typical organisational response to failure is a self-defeating 'vicious circle' of tighter regulation (Johnsson et al., 2014, p.31; Sellman, 2011, p.207; Taleb, 2012). For instance, *The Francis Report* on Mid-Staffordshire NHS Trust found that its board:

> ... did not listen sufficiently to its patients and staff or ensure the correction of deficiencies brought to the Trust's attention. Above all, it failed to tackle an insidious negative culture involving a tolerance of poor standards and a disengagement from managerial and leadership responsibilities. This failure was in part the consequence of allowing a focus on reaching national access targets, achieving financial balance and seeking foundation trust status to be at the cost of delivering acceptable standards of care. (Francis, 2013, p.3)

The inquiry's 290 recommendations contain 390 instances of 'should' and 51 of 'must', many of them examples of tighter control (Raffay, 2016, p.25). Positively, Francis recognised service users might have a role in preventing failure. He suggested 'a set of fundamental standards, easily understood and accepted by patients […] the breach of which will not be tolerated' (Francis, 2013, p.7).

Service users' role in preventing failure has, we suggest, to do with their general preference for value over fact. Forrest and colleagues (2000) found that:

> Many [of the service users interviewed] suggested that nurses who had been educated and professionalized through the hospital-based mental health 'system' ended up perceiving and interacting with users as 'text book cases', rather than individuals with unique experiences of distress. Professional qualities were also seen as eroding the human qualities they valued and this in turn led to 'distance'. (pp.52–53)

Highlighting relationship rather than distance gives internal goods (value) precedence over external goods (fact). It supports the 'art' of nursing, rebalancing evidence-based medicine's preference for outputs or 'science' and preventing Francis's (2013, p.3) 'insidious negative culture' (Moore, 2017; Peplau, 1988). Emphasising the 'art' restates evidence-based medicine's insufficiency. Forrest and colleagues (2000) suggest nurses 'slide up and down the "human" "professional" continuum' in their practice (p. 53). Given nurses (and other clinicians) may experience the 'perfect storm', hardwiring service user preferences into service evaluation might ensure virtuous services (Raffay, 2012b, p.74).

A wider evidence base for evidence-based practice

Ensuring virtuous services requires us to recognise the complexity of organisations. Handy suggests:

> Organizations can be looked at as the fine weave of influence patterns whereby individuals or groups seek to influence others to think or act in

particular ways. If we are to understand organizations we must understand the nature of power and influence for they are the means by which the people of the organisation are linked to its purpose. (Handy, 1993, p.123)

Setting fact over value benefits powerful technocrats and erodes our humanity. Displacing value excludes moral argument other than utilitarianism's dubious circular logic (MacIntyre, 2007, p.56). It favours managers serving the organisation's ends and finds a ready ally in evidence-based medicine's measurable outputs (Moore, 2017, p.109). Evidence-based medicine is liable to bias, and arguably intrinsically biased in rejecting whatever is less quantifiable (Kendall et al., 2011). Thankfully, after Forrest and colleagues' example, we need not discard it. By broadening how we define evidence, we can incorporate value into organisational structures and clinical interactions. In doing so, we deliberately reframe the debate, declaring value necessary.

Salvador-Carulla and colleagues (2017) helpfully propose a 'broader multi-domain perspective' for evidence-based medicine that acknowledges service user experience (p.106). Drawing on systems theory and philosophy of science, they accept that randomised controlled trials devalue experience. They recognise that 'context, expert "opinion" and consumers' experience are factually excluded as relevant sources of knowledge' (p.107). However, in not using a virtue framework, they expose evidence-based medicine's tunnel vision. They suggest scientific knowledge should include: a) observational and experimental evidence based on data; b) contextual knowledge, and c) expert and experiential knowledge (p.110). Significantly, as we clarify in the next section, they suggest this knowledge should be considered from discovery, through collaboration, to implementation. Salvador-Carulla and colleagues' work offers a rationale for moving beyond arguments inspired by antipsychiatry towards exposing the status quo as scientifically and ethically indefensible.

By locating this argument within the fact-value debate, we have revealed vulnerabilities within mental health service provision, suggesting that evidence-based medicine cannot of itself produce happiness. Instead, we have proposed that addressing failure through a self-defeating 'vicious circle' (Johnsson et al., 2014, p.1) of tighter regulation only further weakens the 'broken and demoralised system' (Schizophrenia Commission, 2012, p.3). Virtue approaches, in contrast, prioritise practices that matter to service users and protect against organisational failure. Hardwiring service user preferences into service evaluation and building their experience into the evidence base holds the promise of more effective services.

We started with introducing service user and staff priorities, using the example of spirituality. We then began building a philosophical case for a fresh approach to mental health services. Now, we advance coproduction as the means to achieve this. We propose that services not coproduced from design to evaluation should be considered ethically deficient and that we should establish coproduction as the norm, rather than the exception.

Getting beyond care

We do service users and carers (and staff) an injustice if we only understand their lives relative to mental health services. Further exploration of patient agency puts mental health services in the context of service users' and carers' lives, rather than the other way round. It directs us to address social inequality, discrimination, health promotion and social capital (Swinton, 2000, p.10).

We have suggested that rebalancing with virtue can protect organisations from failure. We have proposed that this is easily achievable by widening the definition of what is acceptable as evidence. We now develop our argument to propose that service users and their carers, and not solely staff, should have a significant say in shaping future mental health services.

Beyond the clinician-patient pairing

In 1988, the UK Government deliberately modelled the NHS on commerce, building the 'perfect storm', and inevitably aligning external goods, bioethics and evidence-based medicine (Griffiths, 1988; Raffay, 2012b). Such an approach clearly conflicts with Kempster and colleagues' (2011, p.322) reflection on Moore's observation (2008, p.499) that, 'The first requirement of a business organization with a virtuous character would be that there is good purpose', and that it is the job of senior managers to ensure this. Within the NHS, the imposition of commercial practices has meant, in MacIntyre's words (2007, p.194), that 'practices could not resist the corrupting power of institutions', with the result that the 'good purpose' is now readily eclipsed by a focus on external goods. Sellman describes how healthcare providers become ensnared:

> Frustratingly, the response to each successive failure of the target culture to deliver on its promises is yet another set of targets with even tighter levels of surveillance leading to ever more severe punishments for failures to meet the targets; a move that encourages ever more unscrupulous behaviour within institutions desperate not to be penalised in the competitive market generated by the league tables that accompany measurement against imposed targets. (Sellman, 2011, p.207)

Kempster and colleagues (2011) suggest effective MacIntyrean leadership can halt this 'inevitable decline' (p.329). However, we believe redesigning the 'broken and demoralised system' through coproduction is likely to be more effective (Schizophrenia Commission, 2012, p.3). Those with lived experience may help us navigate the new territory (Kara, 2013). We may need an active campaign to destigmatise staff with mental health problems, although 'attempts to do so are likely to produce resistance at every level' (May, 2001, p.15).

Redesign, placing the service user rather than profitability centre stage, may be more cost effective. Sullivan proposes that 'patient autonomy is not only a value to guide healthcare but is also the goal of healthcare for chronic disease' (2017, p.13). Rather than lining up external goods, bioethics and evidence-based medicine, coproduction has potential to realign mental health services to service user aspirations. Their hopes provide a powerful value base, offsetting what Kempster and colleagues (2011) saw as 'inevitable decline' (p.329).

Principles of the ethics of coproduction

From the perspective of service users' vital goals, we need an alternative approach to Beauchamp and Childress's *Principles of Biomedical Ethics* (2013) – one that is not centred on clinician agency. Bioethics explores whether the clinician has behaved ethically in the clinical encounter. The ethics of coproduction reunites the 'objectivity–autonomy pairing that radically separates facts from values […] dominant in medical ethics since the Enlightenment' (Sullivan, 2017, p.78). The ethics of coproduction name this divide in mental health services as an artefact of allowing the clinician sole agency (Foucault, 2012). Virtue ethics' commitment to flourishing promises a more fruitful perspective, not least in its recognition of the common good (MacIntyre, 2007; Seedhouse, 2008; Sullivan, 2017). It may be that hope offers a common language between mental health services and faith communities (Kempster et al., 2011; MacIntyre, 2007).

If service users, carers and staff were to work together, based on these principles, we expect the ethics of coproduction would be defined along the following lines. They would:

- begin with the premise that mental health services should be researched, designed, commissioned, delivered and evaluated jointly between service users, carers and staff towards the attainment of common good
- embed virtue through service user, carer and staff experience
- recognise hope as vital
- see all capacitous participants as mutually responsible for outcomes
- understand care as total user experience rather than narrow definitions of treatment

- not be realised through service user and carer representation alone
- not be achieved unless diversity is valued and discrimination mitigated
- envisage departure from these norms as an ethical breach needing clear reasoning, to be considered as a short-term local arrangement, and subject to formal review.

Supremely, the ethics of coproduction are not so much about curing mental illness or even promoting psychological wellbeing. They are about seeking community alongside people with mental health problems in the mainstream community. The vision of such an ethics is social inclusion, which we now consider.

Co-creating wellbeing

Many people with chronic illness experience social exclusion as a more significant burden than their condition (Sullivan, 2017). Swinton argues this may be the case in mental health:

> When we reflect on the life experiences of many people with mental health problems, we find individuals who have to struggle with psychological difficulties that are frequently destructive, incapacitating, and soul-destroying. However, such difficulties are only the beginning of the story of their life struggles. Running alongside the biological and psychological history of people with mental health problems is a form of social experience that is fundamentally degrading, exclusionary, and frequently dehumanizing. When we look into the social experience of people with mental health problems, we discover a level of oppression, prejudice, exclusion, and injustice that is deeply concerning. Negative media images, powerful stigmatizing forces, and exclusion from basic sources of value are just some of the negative experiences that many people experience on a daily basis, simply because they are diagnosed as having a mental health problem. (Swinton, 2000, p.10)

Mental health services are struggling to preserve, let alone improve the nation's mental health, and even the Royal College of Psychiatrists has recognised the need for a new approach (Foley, 2013, p.3). The ethics of coproduction may challenge both mental health services and faith communities to move beyond biomedical and recovery models. Rather than treatment or care – except in emergencies – service users might consider efforts better spent in combatting stigma and securing employment (or other occupation) (Barnes, 2011; Tyszkowska & Podogrodzka, 2013). Interestingly, Sullivan suggests (2017):

> ... autonomy enhancement and the internalization of behavior change are better addressed in educational theory and classical virtue ethics than in theories of health behavior change. (p. 202)

If unable to find new inspiration, the 'broken and demoralised system' risks obsolescence (Schizophrenia Commission, 2012, p.3).

Ideally, service users and their carers, and not only staff, would decide future mental health provision. If this sounds far-fetched, Chambers and colleagues (2014) developed an effective method for gaining informed, although delayed, feedback on experiences of detention. Their approach could readily extend to negotiating better responses from mental health services, faith communities and similar organisations.

Anticipating continued austerity and growing demand on services, we have asserted that much of the literature is entrapped in evidence-based medicine and organisational decline. We have argued that coproduction is likely to prove a better safeguard than Kempster and colleagues' MacIntyrean leadership. More significantly, the principles of the ethics of coproduction reach beyond service redesign to consider hope framed within the community. Stigma may be the greatest obstacle to hope, and inclusion might be service users' and carers' greatest desire from mental health service and faith community support (Rotheram & Raffay, 2017). However, that should be their choice. The ethics of coproduction may become a branch of applied ethics – ideally such a development would be decided through consensus by service users, carers and staff.

Conclusion

Through a logical sequence, we have set up the task of the ethics of coproduction as supporting people with mental health problems and their carers towards hope and community. We first explored spirituality in mental health services through the eyes of service users and suggested it was partly a response to the biopsychosocial model. That led us to argue that service users and staff have different priorities, the former preferring the more compassionate approaches practised by faith communities. Drawing on the fact–value divide described by MacIntyre and Moore, we proposed that service user preferences could help prevent mental health services failure. We suggested incorporating value into organisational structure by including user experience within the evidence base. We next introduced coproduction, arguing for it to become the default ethical position. Finally, we have taken the ethics of coproduction beyond mental health services and reframed it – where reasonable –within the broader ambitions of people who use mental health services and their carers, whatever these might be.

We hope and trust that, just as most reasonably minded people reject slavery, child labour and human traffic as quite simply wrong, before long we will soon think similarly of traditionally delivered mental health services. We don't simply want to see coproduction incorporated into services. We call instead for an altogether different kind of service: one that is fundamentally co-designed, coproduced, co-delivered and co-evaluated. Just as Sullivan argues that 'patients seek the ability not just to pursue health, but also to define and produce health' in response to what they want to achieve in life (2017; pp. 369–370), services should equip people with mental health problems and their loved ones to do just that, wherever reasonable and possible. We should not debase ourselves by settling for anything that is built on anything less than virtue ethics' 'concept of human flourishing (*eudaimonia*) as a thick or full notion of genuine happiness, health, integration, and harmony' (Hall, 2011, p.124).

References

Adkin, M. (2004). *The charge: The real reason why the Light Brigade was lost*. Pimlico.

Banicki, K. (2014). Positive. psychology on character strengths and virtues: A disquieting suggestion. *New Ideas in Psychology, 33*, 21–34.

Barker, P.J. (2003). The tidal model: Psychiatric colonization, recovery and the paradigm shift in mental health care. *International Journal of Mental Health Nursing, 12*, 96–102.

Barnes, H. (2011). Does mental illness have a place alongside social and recovery models of mental health in service users' lived experiences? Issues and implications for mental health education. *The Journal of Mental Health Training, Education and Practice, 6*, 65–75.

Beauchamp, T.L. & Childress, J.F. (2013). *Principles of biomedical ethics*. Oxford University Press.

Brennan, D. (2004). A consideration of the social trajectory of psychiatric nursing in Ireland. *Journal of Psychiatric and Mental Health Nursing, 11*, 494–501.

Cameron, W.B. (1963). *Informal sociology: A casual introduction to sociological thinking*. Random House.

Chambers, M., Gallagher, A., Borschmann, R., Gillard, S., Turner, K. & Kantaris, X. (2014). The experiences of detained mental health service users: Issues of dignity in care. *BMC Medical Ethics, 15*, 1–8.

Duncan, B.L., Miller, S.D., Wampold, B.E. & Hubble, M.A. (2010). *The heart and soul of change: Delivering what works in therapy*. American Psychological Association.

Fernandez, A., Sturmberg, J., Lukersmith, S., Madden, R., Torkfar, G., Colagiuri, R. & Salvador-Carulla, L. (2015). Evidence-based medicine: Is it a bridge too far? *Health Research Policy and Systems, 13*, 1–9.

Foley, T. (2013). *Bridging the gap: The financial case for a reasonable rebalancing of health and care resources*. Royal College of Psychiatrists/Centre for Mental Health.

Forrest, S., Risk, I., Masters, H. & Brown, N. (2000). Mental health service user involvement in nurse education: Exploring the issues. *Journal of Psychiatric and Mental Health Nursing, 7*, 51–57.

Foucault, M. (2012). *The birth of the clinic.* Routledge.

Francis, R. (2013). *Report of the Mid-Staffordshire NHS Foundation Trust public inquiry: Executive summary.* The Stationary Office.

Griffiths, S.R. (1988). *Community care: Agenda for action.* The Stationery Office.

Hall, D.E. (2011). The Guild of Surgeons as a tradition of moral enquiry. *Journal of Medicine and Philosophy, 36*, 114–132.

Handy, C. (1993). *Understanding organizations.* Oxford University Press.

Hinings, C.R. & Mauws, M.K. (2006). Organizational morality. In J.M. Bartunek, M.A. Hinsdale & J.F. Keenan (Eds.), *Church ethics and its organizational context: Learning from the sex abuse scandal in the Catholic Church* (pp.115–122). Sheed & Ward.

Johnsson, L., Eriksson, S., Helgesson, G. & Hansson, M.G. (2014). Making researchers moral. *Research Ethics, 10*, 29–46.

Kara, H. (2013). Mental health service user involvement in research: Where have we come from, where are we going? *Journal of Public Mental Health, 12*, 122–135.

Kempster, S., Jackson, B. & Conroy, M. (2011). Leadership as purpose: Exploring the role of purpose in leadership practice. *Leadership, 7*, 317–334.

Kendall, T., Glover, N., Taylor, C. & Pilling, S. (2011). Quality, bias and service user experience in healthcare: 10 years of mental health guidelines at the UK National Collaborating Centre for Mental Health. *International Review of Psychiatry, 23*, 342–351.

King's Fund. (2011). *The patient-centred care project: Evaluation report.* The King's Fund.

Kitwood, T.M. (1997). *Dementia reconsidered: The person comes first.* Open University Press.

MacIntyre, A. (2007). *After virtue: A study in moral theory* (3rd ed.). Duckworth.

May, R. (2001). Crossing the 'them and us' barriers: An inside perspective on user involvement in clinical psychology. *Clinical Psychology Forum, 150*, 14–17.

Moore, G. (2008). Re-imagining the morality of management: A modern virtue ethics approach. *Business Ethics Quarterly, 18*(4): 483–511.

Moore, G. (2017). *Virtue at work: Ethics for individuals, managers and organizations.* Oxford University Press.

Peplau, H. (1988). The art and science of nursing: Similarities, differences, and relations. *Nursing Science Quarterly, 1*, 8–15.

Raffay, J. (2012a). *What are the factors that prevent or enable the development of a spiritual assessment tool in mental health and that stand in the way of or facilitate the provision of quality spiritual care?* [Unpublished master's.] Cardiff University.

Raffay, J. (2012b). Are our mental health practices beyond HOPE? *Journal of Health Care Chaplaincy, 12*, 68–80.

Raffay, J. (2016). The Francis report (2013): Neo-pharisaism in the NHS? *Health and Social Care Chaplaincy, 4*, 20–34.

Raffay, J., Wood, E. & Todd, A. (2016). Service user views of spiritual and pastoral care (chaplaincy) in NHS mental health services: A co-produced constructivist grounded theory investigation. *BMC Psychiatry, 16*, 200.

Rotheram, C. & Raffay, J. (2017). The life rooms: An innovative recovery approach. *Journal of Recovery in Mental Health, 1*(1), 35–41.

Salvador-Carulla, L., Lukersmith, S. & Sullivan, W. (2017). From the EBM pyramid to the Greek temple: A new conceptual approach to guidelines as implementation tools in mental health. *Epidemiology and Psychiatric Sciences, 26,* 105–114.

Schizophrenia Commission. (2012). *The abandoned illness: A report from the Schizophrenia Commission: Main report.* Schizophrenia Commission.

Seedhouse, D. (2008). *Ethics: The heart of health care.* Wiley.

Sellman, D. (2011). Professional values and nursing. *Medical Health Care and Philosophy, 14,* 203–208.

Slay, J. & Stephens, L. (2013). *Co-production in mental health: A literature review.* New Economics Foundation.

Sullivan, M.D. (2017). *The patient as agent of health and health care.* Oxford University Press.

Swinton, J. (2000). *Resurrecting the person: Friendship and the care of people with mental health problems.* Abingdon Press.

Taleb, N. (2012). *Anti-fragile: How to live in a world we don't understand.* Allen Lane.

Tyszkowska, M. & Podogrodzka, M. (2013). Stigmatization on the way to recovery in mental illness: The factors directly linked to psychiatric therapy. *Psychiatria Polska, 47,* 1011–1022.

Walsh, J., Mcsherry, W. & Kevern, P. (2013). The representation of service users' religious and spiritual concerns in care plans. *Journal of Public Mental Health, 12,* 153–164.

Wonders, S. (2011). *The experiences of those providing pastoral care in the Christian Church community: Supporting people with their mental health and interacting with health professionals.* [Unpublished doctoral thesis.] University of Sheffield.

Chapter 13

Coproducing democratic relationships

Mick McKeown, Albert Dzur and Pamela Fisher

Mental healthcare has rightly been criticised for tendencies to disempower and silence the people who receive its services. Much of this critique concerns the more or less absolute collapse of democratic relations that results from legitimated systems of compulsion and coercion. Notwithstanding this rather obvious point, there is a legacy of broader democratic and institutionalising deficits within mental healthcare that are not always explicable in terms of these overarching psychiatric powers. Such failings often occur at the level of relationships.

Furthermore, it may be the case that deficiencies of democracy in wider society contribute to the existential crises that might cause people to come under the gaze of mental health services in the first place (Fisher, 2009). We live in an epoch of great uncertainty (Bauman, 2000), provoking anxiety and distress that proliferate, alongside the aftermath of trauma in people's lives, to generate the demand for mental health services (Sweeney et al., 2018). In these times, when truth itself is vulnerable and democracy appears to be in crisis, we could be seen to exist on the edge of an advance of authoritarianism and the concentration of power with the few, not the many. Similarly, mental healthcare faces its own legitimacy crisis amidst entrenchment of compulsion and coercion under austerity's squeeze on resources.

Yet, a revitalisation of faith in democracy and renewal of democratic practices is possible, in wider society and in psychiatry. Such democratisation is the promise of coproduction and can be supported even within the most restrictive environments.

Arguably, democratic relationships and processes of coproduction go together neatly. It is hard to conceive of anything that is coproduced that does not result from democratised social relations among the people involved. Similarly, if authentic coproduction takes place, then it must build and strengthen democratic relationships between participants. Thus, democratised relationships are both a means and a consequence of coproduction done properly.

In the mental health services context, the building and strengthening of democratic relations holds the promise of improved experiences and outcomes for service users and a transformed professional identity for providers of care. Democratic professionals acknowledge radical critique of the disenfranchising effects of professional power and aim to work collaboratively with service users, whose agency and knowledge is fully respected and brought to bear in often open-ended processes of cooperative problem-solving (Dzur, 2008, 2017, 2019).

In this chapter, we explore which organisational forms are most likely to support democratised care. First, it is important to locate more recent thinking in a historical and social context. While recognising that any brief historical account will always be inadequate, we turn now to briefly review the impetus for democratising mental healthcare and how, over time, this has occasionally erupted in pointed critique of the mainstream or been realised in situated examples of alternatives.

Tracking democratic tendencies in psychiatry

Long before even the birth of psychiatry as a branch of medicine, people experiencing mental distress have had a need to make their voice heard. Psychiatry was born within the asylum system, and for a while struggled to gain respect among other, more established fields of medicine. The 19th-century growth of asylums and psychiatric practice went hand in hand with a silencing and segregation of individuals deemed to be mad – 'lunatics', in the parlance of the time. Despite variations in the asylums, with relatively more benign care on offer in places such as The Retreat in York, this was an age of incarceration and denial of personal agency. Almost from the start, however, there have been advocates for better care and conditions, and these critical voices and evangelists for change can be tracked forward to our current systems of advocacy and service user involvement, self-organised groups and survivor activism and, latterly, the impulse for coproduction.

Following the Second World War, pioneering practitioners such as Thomas Main, Wilfred Bion and Maxwell Jones began to develop the ideas and practice of therapeutic communities – a distinctly democratic and relational form of care. Key nursing figures such as Annie Altschul and Eileen Skellern were integral to these developments, forming a critical turn in the historical development of modern mental health nursing (Winship et al., 2009). Though few therapeutic communities remain, supporters of the ideal have attempted to hold onto key principles and ensure that these become features of all mental health settings.

In the 1960s and 1970s, a surge in critique of institutionalising mental healthcare and public scandals regarding abuse collided with a noisy (so-called) antipsychiatry movement, populated by, among others, Foucault, Goffman, Szasz and Laing. This energy culminated in a number of progressive developments, not least the long-drawn-out process of closing the asylums and turning towards community care. Such developments were reflected in popular culture, notably Ken Kesey's novel *One Flew Over the Cuckoo's Nest* (Kesey, 1962), which was made into the critically acclaimed film directed by Milos Forman, and more personal, activist-inspired contributions such as Kate Millett's *The Loony Bin Trip* (Millett, 1990). R.D. Laing and David Cooper combined a counter-cultural critique of wider society with psychiatry to develop a form of therapeutic community that culminated in the Philadelphia Association community houses, including Kingsley Hall.

Groups such as the Mental Patients Union in the 1970s and, later, Survivors Speak Out and Mad Pride in the 1980s and 1990s, represented a determined effort at self-organisation and reclaiming the right to be heard in one's own voice. Interestingly, the English wing of the Mental Patients' Union (MPU) emerged out of struggles to defend Paddington Day Hospital, an outpatient therapeutic community. This suggests that radical service user activism and associated alliances with critical professionals were able to thrive in an already democratised setting (Spandler, 2006). Such social movement organisations have waxed and waned over the years but have always had a critical and influential presence. Latterly, newer groups are organising themselves using social media, including activists allied to Mad Studies and Recovery in the Bin.[1]

The great scholar and activist for socialist and mental health transformations, Peter Sedgwick, who also worked in the therapeutic community at Grendon Underwood prison, published *Psycho Politics* in 1982. This is a book that is still relevant today (Cresswell & Spandler, 2009; Proctor, 2016; Spandler et al., 2016). Sedgwick offered a searing critique of the antipsychiatry arguments for neglecting to engage with mental health as a political idea. For Sedgwick, to be against psychiatry and not argue for something credible in its place, was ultimately an act of political conservatism. So, Sedgwick argued for 'more and

---

1. www.recoveryinthebin.org

better psychiatry'. But, for him, this was to be framed around democratic and relational ideals, and alternative approaches conceived in a 'prefigurative politics' – shaping the world we would like to see in the act of trying to bring it about. To achieve this, Sedgwick argued for cross-sectional alliances between service users, their family carers, professionals and social movements.

Such alternative forms of mental healthcare have emerged from time to time in the historical record or can be glimpsed in the different ways in which practitioners and service users occasionally adapt or subvert practice in the mainstream by opening up spaces for intruding more democracy or compassion into everyday relationships of care. In this regard, Spandler (2009, p.672) speaks of 'spaces of psychiatric contention' and Crossley (1999, p.809) identifies exemplar 'working utopias'. Perhaps more radically, user-led, non-medical alternatives have similarly been developed in the face of a perceived intransigence to change on the part of the mainstream and associated mistrust of the clinical workforce (Russo & Sweeney, 2016).

Emerging partly from the seeds of some of the antipsychiatry critique and a personal revulsion at the dehumanising effects of institutional services, Franco Basaglia started the Psichiatria Democratica (Democratic Psychiatry) movement in Italy, campaigning for legal reforms that would ultimately close their asylums, in a move away from institutional care. Although there were undoubtedly some mixed results for service users, 'this movement was a struggle for liberation, for democracy and for equality' and does not deserve much of the negative appraisal it received at the hands of historians of mainstream psychiatry (Foot, 2014, p.245). Basaglia's advocacy directly influenced activists in the UK, inspiring the establishment of *Asylum: The Magazine for Democratic Psychiatry* in 1986 (now renamed *Asylum: The radical mental health magazine*).

The territory of seeking change within psychiatry and society is occupied by service users, refusers, survivors and critically minded people who work in psychiatry. It is also possible for staff to share experience of mental ill health, not least because mental health services, especially under austerity, can be stressful places to work in, and the structures and processes that alienate patients can also be alienating for staff. This can especially be the case for staff who prefer not to take up an oppressive role, which arguably the overwhelming majority do not, yet find themselves operating an increasingly coercive system, despite the shift to community care. Many mental health workers are also members of radical groups seeking more democratic and consensual services, including groups such as the Critical Psychiatry Network, the Social Work Action Network and the Critical Mental Health Nurses Network. A democratic professionalism affords one means to escape staff experiences of alienation and extend consciousness raising across teams and staff groups.

Sedgwick aligned himself clearly to democratic political activism but bemoaned the lack of preparedness on the political left. With the existence of radical service user and staff constituencies, a productive place to start would be alliances for change between worker trade unions and survivor groupings (McKeown et al., 2014). The craft of building such solidarity has, to date, arguably been imperfect, risking reinventing the sort of power imbalances that exist in services. That said, the desire for more equal, relational, democratic services could be the basis for shaping such aspects within fledgling alliances, with a coming together of therapeutic and activist ideals of democracy, communication and relationships. The fact that trade unions face their own legitimacy crisis and many are attempting to solve this by programmes of democratic renewal offers some promise for re-establishing more reciprocal relations with communities and wider social movements. To lay the foundations for helpful alliances, we may require reparative processes for healing the previous harms inflicted by psychiatric care (Spandler & McKeown, 2017).

Democracy at large

Public intellectuals such as Jurgen Habermas and Pierre Rosanvallon (2008) in Europe and John Rawls in the US have made a case for more deliberative, democratic processes in the public domain. The emphasis is placed on dialogue, rather than individuals thinking in private about voting choices. Instead, these forms of democracy involve reasoned and reasonable communication between many people, in a curious, creative collective of voices. Those who participate must respect each other, regardless of difference, and attempt to work equally, despite any existing privileges or power differences. Ideally, enough time is taken for discussion and debate, with participants attempting to persuade each other to particular points of view while simultaneously remaining open to changing their own minds.

Feminist, disability and other movement actors have modified these ideas to allow for the fact that powerful emotions may be present, and any democracy has to create a space that can hold this, maintain respect for others, and move forward without falling apart (Young, 1996). In this vein, critical voices allied to survivor movements who link the personal with the political have spoken of the turbulent communication that can arise in the context of attempting to change mental health services and policies (Church, 1995). From this perspective, the rebellious and recalcitrant contribution may have more legitimacy in the quest for meaningful change than the meekly co-operative stance, which can be too readily co-opted to the continuance of the status quo (McKeown, 2016). So, we may have what the Canadian sociologist Michael Gardiner (2004) has called 'wild publics', as much as polite, civilised, largely middle-class debates.

The proliferation of a range of ostensibly democratic spaces and opportunities for civic engagement can be seen as both a blessing and a curse for activists committed to substantive social change. With a generalised loss of faith in electoral democracy and the institutions of government and welfare, there is an ever-present hazard for community actors of co-option and dilution of impact. If this results in further erosion of trust in democracy, then all the better for neoliberal power. Despite such challenges, authentic and meaningfully democratic civic action can and does take place, and can be strengthened by remaining alert to the various hazards, criticisms and subtle lapses that can undermine the mobilisation of activist resources towards goals of real social change (Dzur, 2019).

The co-operative and relational aspects of deliberative democracy can deliver higher-quality decisions or resolve conflict and, ultimately, serve an educative purpose – helping people to become more civically orientated and promote greater collective affinity for civic virtues. Such civic action usually coalesces around an agreed unity of purpose, often located within distinct neighbourhoods facing particular challenges. In recognising this, we should perhaps not lose sight of the forms of deliberation that take place in the everyday, which may lack the unity of purpose that underpins organised systems of deliberation. This everyday communication, regardless of occasional antagonisms or lack of co-operation and agreement, can nevertheless also be a vehicle for realising civic virtues. For example, it is possible for good communicators to begin a deliberative process from adversarial positions and still achieve good decisions or resolution of problems (Hutton Ferris, 2019).

Dissent, resistance and recalcitrance, however boisterously communicated, are also legitimate expressions of democratic will. A new politics of mental health must accommodate the full range of voices on the mental health territory, from co-operators to dissidents. Doing justice to this will allow for new, alternative forms of care to emerge and begin to dissolve false 'us and them' distinctions between staff and service users, refusers and survivors, while doing justice to real differences and the tangible realities of mental distress. For Sedgwick (1982), the way we must change psychiatry is to forge, at scale, better human relationships in our response to this distress.

These relational goals are also, arguably, the best way to transform society as a whole, in a quest for a more equal, democratic world. Commentators such as Rex Haigh, steeped in the heritage of therapeutic communities but concerned with wider social import and change, have argued for improved understanding of the relational basis of all human development (Haigh & Benefield, 2019). Similarly, others have pointed out the huge importance of forms of place and space to better support healing and recovery from both interpersonal and societally inflicted trauma (see Chapter 5, this volume). Hence, we require attention to all such factors in conceiving of both the form and process of democratised care and support. It is to some of the available forms of democratic practices within mental healthcare that we now turn.

Democracy in coproduction

Mental health services and society can be as injurious to individuals' sense of themselves as legitimate citizens as they are felt to be helpful or supportive of recovery. Key social and psychiatric forces conspire to undermine personal agency, hope and self-belief, and, despite all the rhetoric about empowerment, are thus deeply disempowering (Fisher, 2016). As this very fact becomes apparent to a wider public, it forms the basis for the legitimacy crisis facing psychiatry. However, simultaneously, it can also be the basis for constructive, cross-sectional alliances for change, including those that are forged between service users and professionals.

Coproduction as an ideal arrives in the policy rhetoric of mental health services, following numerous previous flag carriers for democratisation, such as service user involvement and shared decision-making. These have delivered notable democratic gains alongside more sobering failings to meaningfully transform routine care. The failings have often resulted from a dissonance between the talk about empowerment and disempowerment and a real lack of serious thought and engagement with the actualities of iniquitous power distribution. If coproduction as a strategic goal is not to repeat the same mistakes, then prevailing power differentials and the respective positionings of the various protagonists must be addressed head on (Stacey et al., 2016). Deliberative democratic communication holds promise for navigating these constraints, but can also be rendered impotent in the face of organisations unwilling to surrender power or trapped in the neoliberal vices of privatisation and new public management.

Thus, democracy in mental healthcare becomes more than just the adoption of systems for paying attention to voice and choice. The Open Dialogue approach emerging out of Western Lapland in Finland explicitly draws on Bakhtin's theories of dialogue (Seikkula & Olson, 2003) to make the case for an unashamedly democratised therapy that results in substantially improved outcomes for service users and their families, while offering more equal and fulfilling working relationships for participating staff. Other such alternatives to simplistic biological psychiatry emphasise, in various ways, the relational over the technical, and, where these have been subject to research, have often demonstrated equivalence with mainstream services' outcomes while using minimal or no medication (Calton et al., 2008).

Critical and radical practitioners in health and social care services need to persuade their colleagues and representative unions of the importance and value of prescriptions for change, and, in so doing, forge constructive alliances to action that are as much informed by survivor voices as by professional or intellectual contributions. The necessary collective dialogue to take us there may well be unsettled and unsettling, but from this can be found more creative and impactful strategies. Getting past turbulent disagreement will undoubtedly require a loving quest for mutual understanding and recognition (Fisher, 2008). To this end, the scholar of disability and care ethics, Marian Barnes (2012), coined the term 'care-full' deliberation to refer to the need for democratic activists to take care of each other in the course of building their movements – a plea that could resonate equally powerfully in the arena of professional caring relationships.

The extent to which conventional professionals working within mainstream psychiatric organisations can achieve the sort of democratic changes in services demanded by service user and survivor social movements is constrained by various factors – not least tensions between their different perspectives. The activists must make serious inroads to persuade more than a few status-quo professionals, and these professionals must be open to persuasion. Many activists are rightly frustrated with institutions and professionals and just want to chisel out what resources they can and create practices and subcultures outside professionalised domains. Conventional professionals, for their part, can distrust activists' politicisation of topics they believe are non-ideological. To have a coproductive meeting of minds requires a special kind of fruitful conflict wherein those holding different standpoints become aware of the strengths of others' positions and the weaknesses of their own. This may prove to be an unstable foundation for coproductive relationships; deliberative processes designed to hold and contain powerful emotional responses without derailing goals become perhaps stretched to breaking point. Recognising this suggests that it ought to be staff who make the first moves to enact democratic change within services.

Notwithstanding such challenges, most practitioners need to overcome numerous other barriers within the systems they work in if they are to assume the mantle of democratic professional. Such constraints include the counter-democratic demands placed on staff by, for instance, bureaucratic systems geared up for effective and efficient control of spending and resources; legislative frameworks that demarcate zones of responsibility and authority, and economically incentivised professional claims for jurisdictional control over particular tasks, issues and problems. Given such constraints, that some not-trivial progress towards the democratisation of professional practice has been realised is testament to the value of the idea of coproduction (Dzur, 2019).

Transforming psychiatry, transforming society

Sedgwick (1982) made the astute observation that the tools and goals for transforming psychiatry are essentially the same as those required for broader social change, and that these are ultimately relational. Moreover, the mental health system and the wider political economy are intimately enmeshed. Mark Fisher (2009) famously noted that it might be easier to imagine the end of the world than to conceive of the demise of capitalism. He also wryly pointed out how certain issues appear to be de-politicised under neoliberal capitalism. For him, mental health is one such example – generally accepted among the wider public, and for that matter, the political left, as an uncomplicated fact rather than being open to political contestation. Yet, paradoxically, growing awareness of epidemics of mental distress suggests that capitalism itself is inherently dysfunctional. Even scholars working in mainstream economics (such as Nobel prize winner Angus Deaton) have drawn attention to the powerful links between capitalism, inequality and what he and his wife Anne Case call 'deaths of despair' (Case & Deaton, 2020). Interestingly, for Fisher (2009, p.80), mental health problems represent forms of 'captured discontent', and an effective political strategy is to realise this and convert such disaffections into action against their root causes within an unfair society.

Where then should we make a start in this dual task of reimagining mental healthcare alongside societal understanding of mental health itself? With relevance for democratic ideals, Taggart (2018) points out the limits of an ethics of rationality in making sense of acts notable for their irrationality or the 'out-of-this-world' experiences of trauma victims. Aware of the potential for purposely therapeutic relationships to risk re-traumatising individuals whose trauma and distress resulted from abusive relationships in the first place, he draws on the philosopher Emmanuel Levinas to propose an ethics of responsibility to other people. Thus, forging a radical and respectful empathy with other people, regardless of their apparent strangeness or irrationality, challenges the objectifying or dehumanising tendencies of categorical or transactional approaches to clinical practice and opens up novel ways of dealing with trauma. Perceiving such relational duties and obligations to the 'other' may also assist us to deepen the quality of our democracies, especially in getting to grips with the need to show respect across difference. This is especially pertinent with regard to people deemed to be mentally ill: the irrational, marginalised and routinely silenced.

Professionals attempting to put coproduction ideals into practice do face certain openings and opportunities that can arise from the contextual, situational and relational complexities of their work. Such opportunities for service transformations can be supported by other openings to mobilise community resources and seek supportive alliances in communities. There are many wicked problems in these professional care contexts (see Hannigan & Coffey, 2011); faced with difficult or even intractable challenges that are impervious to solution from singular perspectives, services can more readily consider collaborative approaches. Hierarchical and risk-averse systems may be more amenable to relaxing their centralised control when more participatory efforts show positive results with no increase in risk. This is achieved first and foremost by harnessing a wider pool of problem-solving knowledge and expertise, particularly that held by users of services and their community allies. All participants in hierarchical systems can come to the realisation that rigid managerialism is the enemy of much curiosity, innovation and progressive change.

As things stand, mental health services and social welfare provision in the UK (and other neoliberal states) are beset with a preoccupation with risk management, risk assessment and risk governance strategies. Members of marginalised social groups are, in this context, stigmatised as the risky 'other'. Risk is limited through a strategy of restricting agency, and loss of agency is in itself a significant aspect of being 'othered'. The loss of agency, experienced most acutely by services users, extends also to professionals who work in environments where opportunities for attentive responsiveness are limited by the demands of risk-assessment practices that may be used as forensic sources for allocating blame when things go wrong. For all these reasons, strategic adoption of more democratic, participatory approaches to getting the job done are urgently needed to provide swifter, more agile and responsive organisational working that better meets people's expressed needs and effectively sustains wellbeing in the process of its enactment (Dzur, 2019).

Conclusions

Returning to Peter Sedgwick's vision for future thinking and action, we can appreciate the case he makes for a democratised psychiatry. Resonance with the appeal of coproduction is clear, but also required is an activist's evaluation of authenticity of implementation and situating mental healthcare within a broader social and political frame. Above all, Sedgwick's attachment to prefigurative practices holds the promise for more compassionate, loving, non-coercive services and the democratic, relational and cooperative means by which these may be realised.

It is a truism on the left that unity is strength; it is a tragedy in equal measure that this solidarity is seldom perfectly achieved. Debates about the future direction of mental health services will be more complete and meaningful with recourse to critical, but subtle, materialist thinking, not least for locating struggles for more and better services within a societal analysis of power and oppression. Sedgwick's genius was to combine such understanding with anarchist ideas for the sort of prefigurative social relations necessary to deliver these ends without reinventing various self-defeating tyrannies along the way or neglecting the importance of the everyday. The world and psychiatric services need a healthy dose of bright, maverick, indignant, kind and comradely resistance; Sedgwick's psychopolitics provide an exemplary blueprint for those of a recalcitrant disposition, heralding a democratisation of mental healthcare and support fit for the 21st century.

A lived coproduction in action may be difficult to achieve, but practitioners who make the effort may find that oppressive systems are 'revisable in ways that cannot be anticipated' (Fisher, 2016, p.346) and the necessary openness can be supported by the development of genuine coproduction processes, making use of the best of relational practice and deliberative democratic ideals.

References

Barnes, M. (2012). *Care in everyday life: An ethic of care in practice*. Policy Press.

Bauman, Z. (2000). *Liquid modernity*. Polity Press.

Calton, T., Ferriter, M., Huband, N. & Spandler, H. (2008). A systematic review of the Soteria paradigm for the treatment of people diagnosed with schizophrenia. *Schizophrenia Bulletin, 34*(1), 181–192.

Case, A. & Deaton, A. (2020). *Deaths of despair and the future of capitalism*. Princeton University Press.

Church, K. (1995). *Forbidden narratives: Critical autobiography as social science*. Routledge.

Cresswell, M. & Spandler, H. (2009). Psychopolitics: Peter Sedgwick's legacy for the politics of mental health. *Social Theory & Health, 7*(2), 129–147.

Crossley, N. (1999). Working utopias and social movements: An investigation using case study materials from radical mental health movements in Britain. *Sociology, 33*(4), 809–830.

Dzur, A.W. (2008). *Democratic professionalism: Citizen participation and the reconstruction of professional ethics, identity, and practice*. Penn State Press.

Dzur, A.W. (2017). *Rebuilding public institutions together: Professionals and citizens in a participatory democracy*. Cornell University Press.

Dzur, A.W. (2019). *Democracy inside: Participatory innovation in unlikely places*. Oxford University Press.

Fisher, M. (2009). *Capitalist realism: Is there no alternative?* Zero Books.

Fisher, P. (2008). Wellbeing and empowerment: The importance of recognition. *Sociology of Health & Illness, 30*(4), 583–598.

Fisher, P. (2016). Coproduction: What is it and where do we begin? *Journal of Psychiatric and Mental Health Nursing, 23*, 345–346.

Foot, J. (2014). Franco Basaglia and the radical psychiatry movement in Italy, 1961–78. *Critical and Radical Social Work, 2*(2), 235–249.

Gardiner, M.E. (2004). Wild publics and grotesque symposiums: Habermas and Bakhtin on dialogue, everyday life and the public sphere. *The Sociological Review, 52*(s1), 28–48.

Haigh, R. & Benefield, N. (2019). Towards a unified model of human development. *Mental Health Review Journal, 24*(2), 124–132.

Hannigan, B. & Coffey, M. (2011). Where the wicked problems are: The case of mental health. *Health Policy, 101*(3), 220–227.

Hutton Ferris, D. (2019). Civic virtue in the deliberative system. *Journal of Public Deliberation, 15*(1), 6. www.publicdeliberation.net/jpd/vol15/iss1/art6

Kesey, K. (1962). *One flew over the cuckoo's nest.* Viking.

McKeown, M. (2016). Stand up for recalcitrance! *International Journal of Mental Health Nursing, 25*, 481–483.

McKeown, M., Cresswell, M. & Spandler, H. (2014). Deeply engaged relationships: Alliances between mental health workers and psychiatric survivors in the UK. In B. Burstow, B. LeFrancois & S. Diamond (Eds.), *Psychiatry disrupted: Theorizing resistance and crafting the revolution* (pp.193–216). McGill/Queen's University Press.

Millett, K. (1990). *The looney bin trip.* Simon & Schuster.

Proctor, H. (2016). Lost minds: Sedgwick, Laing and the politics of mental illness. *Radical Philosophy, 197*(May/June), 36–48.

Rosanvallon, P. (2008). *Counter-democracy: Politics in an age of distrust.* Cambridge University Press.

Russo, J. & Sweeney, A. (2016). Introduction. In J. Russo & A. Sweeney (Eds.), *Searching for a rose garden: Challenging psychiatry, fostering mad studies* (pp.1–5). PCCS Books.

Sedgwick, P. (1982). *Psycho politics.* Pluto Press.

Seikkula, J. & Olson, M.E. (2003). The open dialogue approach to acute psychosis: Its poetics and micropolitics. *Family Process, 42*(3), 403–418.

Spandler, H. (2006). *Asylum to action: Paddington day hospital, therapeutic communities and beyond.* Jessica Kingsley Publishers.

Spandler, H. (2009). Spaces of psychiatric contention: A case study of a therapeutic community. *Health & Place, 15*(3), 672–678.

Spandler, H. & McKeown, M. (2017). Exploring the case for truth and reconciliation in mental health. *Mental Health Review Journal, 22*(2), 83–94.

Spandler, H., Moth, R., McKeown, M. & Greener, J. (2016). Psychopolitics in the twenty first century. *Critical and Radical Social Work, 4*(3), 307–312.

Stacey, G., Felton, A., Morgan, A., Stickley, T., Willis, M., Diamond, B., Houghton, P., Johnson, B. & Dumenya, J. (2016). A critical narrative analysis of shared decision-making in acute inpatient mental health care. *Journal of Interprofessional Care, 30*(1), 35–41.

Sweeney, A., Filson, B., Kennedy, A., Collinson, L. & Gillard, S. (2018). A paradigm shift: Relationships in trauma-informed mental health services. *BJPsych Advances, 24*(5), 319–333.

Taggart, D. (2018). Trauma and an ethics of responsibility. *Clinical Psychology Forum, 302*, 4–14.

Winship, G., Bray, J., Repper, J. & Hinshelwood, R.D. (2009). Collective biography and the legacy of Hildegard Peplau, Annie Altschul and Eileen Skellern: The origins of mental health nursing and its relevance to the current crisis in psychiatry. *Journal of Research in Nursing, 14*(6), 505–517.

Young, I.M. (1996). Inclusion and the other: Beyond deliberative democracy. In S. Benhabib (Ed.), *Democracy and difference: Contesting the boundaries of the political* (pp.120–135). Princeton University Press.

Coproducing the future: Conclusion

Don Bryant

In this section, we have seen the benefits and justification for coproduction as well as problems getting it widely acclaimed. I must admit to a certain disappointment that the practice of coproduction has not advanced as quickly or as universally as I would have hoped. Back in 2013, Mind, the UK mental health charity, engaged the New Economics Foundation (NEF) to appraise coproduction (Slay & Stephens, 2013). NEF reviewed 15 successful coproduction projects, across the country, hoping to:

> ... reinvigorate interest and commitment to co-production in the commissioning, design, delivery and evaluation of services, in order to truly transform services across all mental health settings. We know that much has been done already in this area but there is much more to do before coproduction becomes the norm. (Slay & Stephens, 2013, p.1)

By 2016, the National Development Team for inclusion (NDTi) published *Embedding Co-production in Mental Health: A framework for strategic leads, commissioners and managers*. This offered a supporting structure for enacting coproduction – in essence, a policy and procedures document only needing minor amendments to fit individual organisational requirements. They concluded:

> If coproduction in mental health is to lead to meaningful and sustainable change, it has to be embedded within and across systems and reflected in how professionals and service users, their carers and groups come together, as equals, valuing each others' skills, strengths and expertise.

> Leaders have a critical role to play in setting the right culture and conditions in which co-production takes root and becomes 'the way in which things are done around here'. Paying close attention to the cultural and behavioural changes required will help to create lasting change and should lead to better outcomes for people who use mental health services, their families, friends, organisations, communities and the wider system, as well as confident staff who are empowered to work co-productively. (NDTi, 2016, p.4)

Looking forward, the blog *The Rise of Coproduction: Benefits, opportunities and challenges* (Hodgkinson et al., 2016, p.1) asked:

> So what does the future hold for co-production? Will we see an upsurge in the use of coproduction as researchers and policy makers recognise its worth and seek to improve the relevance of their work? Or will the ambiguity and challenges put people off from using these methods? It is clear that – when employed thoughtfully – co-production has the potential to revolutionise particular forms of research and service design. However, to ensure co–production delivers benefits to those who have been catered to least, there is clearly a need for significant new skills, resources and commitment to a different way of working.

This emphasises the virtues of coproduction, but also acknowledges challenges and difficulties. Despite growing talk and interest around coproduction, arguably there are too few authentic examples in practice and no cohesive national structure. Why is this?

Some contributing factors that impede the necessary openness and democracy for coproduction to gain traction include:

- There is immense staff fatigue around new initiatives and change. We have seen workloads increase for all NHS professionals, partly due to vastly decreased staffing and the never-ending insistence on providing data and recording output (often for little obvious purpose). Therefore, there can be resistance to new ideas which demand time to implement.
- Risk-averse systems operate on a hierarchical basis that at times leads to inertia.
- The degree of autonomy of the individual mental health trusts in England might explain variability in implementation of coproduction. A creeping culture of competition rather than cooperation can be the enemy of communication and coordination.

- Internal and public-facing communications, such as glossy magazines, tend to be one-way, with trusts passing down selected information and 'good news' dominating, rather than encouraging constructive debate around challenges, deficits or new possibilities.

At the beginning of 2018, my local NHS provider made a decision to discontinue a service that directly affected some 200 service users. The decision was made without consultation and communicated as a *fait accompli*. The decision was explained as 'cost-cutting', due to budgetary constraints. I wrote to the board of directors to question the manner in which the decision had been made, without service user representation or alternative provision. This was discussed by the board. The chief executive, whom I greatly respect and admire, replied. Reportedly, as the financial information was deemed 'sensitive', they could not include service users in their decision. It is likely I would have received the same response from the vast majority, if not all, mental health trusts. Here lies the problem: is it an issue of trust – that service users might not respect confidentiality? Is it that senior managers and staff would be disgruntled if service users knew information they did not? Is it an expression of power? Or is it that 'this is the way it has always been done'? Whichever, the lack of transparency and democracy is exposed.

During the past 10 years, fellow service users, carers and I have discussed the best approach to remedy some of the above. Should we try and influence the board of directors and, with their authority, feed coproduction ideals down through the organisation? Do we start at the bottom, in small, often discrete groups, and hope that successes will be passed upwards? The answer is probably both, although it would be much quicker if we had the impetus and influence from above.

Despite setbacks, I remain optimistic that coproduction will become an everyday part of health provision, but this may very well take time. That will not stop me and many other like-minded people from trying to accelerate the process and to convert influential decision-makers to join forces with us. We have the knowledge, motivation and expertise to democratise mental health services. Understanding challenges and impediments is important but we should avoid being demoralised by past experiences by keeping in view a more progressive vision for the future. We should learn the lessons of the past and avoid repeating mistakes.

References

Hodgkinson, S., Rimmer, M. & Salway, S. (2016). *The rise of co-production: Benefits, opportunities and challenges.* Public Health Topics.

National Development Team for Inclusion (NDTi) (2016). *Embedding co-production in mental health: A framework for strategic leads, commissioners and managers.* National Development Team for Inclusion.

Slay, J. & Stephens, L. (2013). *Co-production in mental health: A literature review.* New Economics Foundation.

Conclusions

David Pilgrim

Attempts at definitions of coproduction made by the contributors to this book locate it as a public policy aspiration with positive intentions emerging in the late 20th century. The efficiency of services might improve; this follows the logic of all service industries that use feedback on consumer satisfaction about current provision and user advice about what is being planned. The client's position as an active agent and citizen might be better respected; this follows the spirit of liberal democracies to provide recognition to us all as human beings (Alford, 2009; Honneth, 1995). These offers seem both eminently sensible and democratic in character, and so it would be churlish to reject them out of hand.

However, those positive intentions, as many of the contributors note, are constrained or even negated by other processes. Professional power is highly adaptive and might incorporate reforms, such as those based on coproduction. That incorporation or 'co-option' might then erode or even reverse the cause of individual and collective client empowerment. Moreover, what if the latter is genuinely limited by impaired client potential and functioning? In a modern, complex world governed by the principle of rationality, those who are deemed to have lost their reason (or, in the case of those with learning disabilities, where it is less developed) are at a disadvantage at the outset.

Moreover, concerns with system efficiency and consumer involvement have emerged for reasons other than a democratic and humanistic sensibility about the end-point recipients of health and social care; they also reflect to some extent the contradictions of the welfare state. Welfare clients are poor and a burden on state expenditure, and yet the health and welfare systems contain the distress, dysfunction and consequent social disruption created by modern capitalism. Accordingly, the latter cannot live with the welfare state but also cannot live without it (Offe, 1993).

The notion of active citizens at liberty in society was promoted by J.S. Mill, but he also argued that exceptions should apply in relation to children, 'idiots' and 'lunatics'. That is the very reason why old-fashioned professional paternalism seemed to be readily warranted and 'mental health law' accrued a reputation for being socially progressive, obscuring its routine and actual function of justifying coercive social control. The notion of 'care', for example, sounds positive: if we are looked after benignly by those 'in the know', then we might be grateful and we might truly benefit from being the passive recipients of expertise. Good professionals, like good parents, might offer genuinely good care for their fellows. However, if there is a bringing together, as there is in 'mental health policy', between care and control, then these basic assumptions can become obscured (Cohen & Scull, 1983).

The imperative of paternalistic care and its potential advantage proved to be highly problematic when health and social services emerged in industrial societies in the 19th century, and were subsequently consolidated in developed economies. In that modern social context, sociologists following Durkheim, who studied professionals, certainly endorsed their positive social value and respected their scarce knowledge and expertise. However, those following Weber proved to be far more distrustful about the power asymmetries created by professionals, with Marxians being confused as to whether they were part of the proletariat or agents of the state acting on behalf of the ruling class (Macdonald, 1995).

Apart from professionals pursuing their own interests at the expense of their clients, they might also at times be ineffective in their efforts and even injurious. The neglect and abuse of inpatients in isolated systems by professionals exercising their self-interested power persisted in the 20th century (Martin, 1985). At the centre of this problem was a lack of trust. Politicians and policymakers could not always trust professionals to be effective and humane. Clients in turn could not always trust professionals to be 'kindly and efficacious', to use a term still relevant today and offered at the end of the 'antipsychiatry' period by Sedgwick (1982).

One strategy to guard against these threats to trust from both policymakers and end-point users of services was to incorporate the client perspective in a range of ways; coproduction is the most recent iteration. It contains within it the historically accrued contradictions of the good intentions of state paternalism ('*parens patriae*') alongside the episodic scandalous failings of professionalised forms of care. One metaphor then is that it is a 'curate's egg'. Another might be that it is a cork bobbing on choppy water made turbulent by conflicts between interest groups (Alford, 1975). Unpacking these metaphors, we find the expressed ambivalence of the social actors involved in situated efforts at coproduction, as well as ambiguities within the social contexts of those efforts.

Ambivalence and ambiguity

If it is obvious in the preceding chapters that a range of social actors are implicated in promoting or constraining coproduction and other client-centred and consumerist initiatives in the welfare state, then it is also obvious that wider contextual features that are supra-personal can and should be examined. The human agents involved, with their varying collective and individual expectations, are part of the picture about coproduction. Their ambivalence bears examination, but so too does their embedding context. The latter preceded their existence and may impact in ways that are not obvious to people (be they professionals or clients). Elsewhere, I have adopted the philosophical resource of critical realism to explore this interaction of epistemological relativism (the range of views held by social actors) and ontological realism (the material and ideological forces affecting those actors) in relation to mental health (Pilgrim, 2015).

Ambivalence from the actors involved in promoting or impeding coproduction is evident. This can be seen at the collective level (the demands of interest groups) and individually. Policymakers are ambivalent about the direction of mental health policy because they are constantly balancing the implied or expressed needs of end-point users with those who are sane by common consent. For example, the efficiency of a service at tidying up risky scenarios in everyday life can be contrasted with the acceptability of that service to identified patients. Being sectioned under the Mental Health Act resolves a social crisis (all mental health crises are social crises), but it is at the expense of the identified patient, who loses their liberty without trial and may endure unwanted bodily interference that is deemed now to be care, not assault (Bean, 1980). This tension about balancing interests has also been evident in relation to community treatment orders, so this is not only about inpatient admission (Fabris, 2011; Riley et al., 2018).

At the same time, policymakers in late modernity have a wider commitment to consumerism for reasons of hoped-for improvements in efficiency and the promotion of a humane service ideology. The shift in emphasis from coercion to voluntarism in the early 20th century exemplifies this point. In Britain until 1930, *all* patients were detained involuntarily. However, policymakers to this day have not taken the full step of abandoning coercive 'mental health' legislation. This is a clear signal that relying on voluntary action remains carefully contained by higher-order political requirements: the state's need to ensure social control of the population when and if required. Mental health professionals provide that function.

When we turn to the ambivalence of mental health professionals, this mirrors the policymakers' dilemma. How can care as an emotional desire, not just a set of codified, skilled practices, be held centre stage at all times? How are third-party demands from those sane by common consent to be dealt with? One professional response has been to embrace the paternalistic commitment to treat mentally ill people, whether or not the latter request it; psychiatric care then is an *ethical obligation* that overrides the expressed needs of patients. Complete paternalism may be simplistic in its moral justification, but it is at least consistent. That position was mainly adopted by biodeterminists in the Kraepelinian tradition.

Unreflective and complete paternalism also comes to the relief of those who are sane by common consent, as they are content to leave to the psychiatric profession the resolution of some sorts of social-existential crisis in life. Loss of liberty and coercive interference are defensible in the public imagination; they are the price worth paying to maintain social order and a sense of daily personal security. An underlying doubt remains, though, because the main fear the public has about psychiatry and its coercive powers is that of 'unfair detention'. Expectations that professionals should always offer optimal care in exchange for loss of liberty (the 'principle of reciprocity') have failed to be fulfilled for the very reason that humane care and the pragmatics of control are inherently poor bedfellows (Eastman, 1994). If psychiatric care is so good, then why must it be imposed at times and why is it feared so much by the prospective patient?

However, Kraepelinian psychiatry and its taken-for-granted paternalism and biomedical routines has only been one, albeit a dominant, expression in professional training and clinical routines. For example, one reading of the history of the *Diagnostic and Statistical Manual of Mental Disorders* (American Psychiatric Association, 2013) has been of an unstable and revisable outcome of ideological tensions between three factions within the American Psychiatric Association (APA): the biodeterminists, the psychoanalysts and the social psychiatrists. It is hardly surprising, then, that the libertarian leaders of 'antipsychiatry' after the Second World War were psychoanalysts (Laing, 1966; Szasz, 1963). It is also not surprising that the social psychiatric tradition traceable in the main to the work of Adolf Meyer in Baltimore in the 1930s gave confidence to many psychiatrists to displace diagnoses with more holistic biopsychosocial formulations (Double, 2007; Engel, 1980) and to argue for compassionate, person-centred care as an alternative to paternalism.

Thus, the psychiatric profession has been divided over the matter of paternalism and has at times been at the forefront of reforms to services to render them both 'kindly and efficacious' (Pilgrim, 2018). One expression of those reforms has been a regard for both client-centred negotiations in clinical routines, which respect biographical uniqueness, and an emphasis on social overview, not just clinical insight. Those outside of or in opposition to the Kraepelinian tradition have thereby encouraged client-centred negotiations to mitigate professional paternalism. This has been part of the space created for the theory and practice of coproduction to emerge in the field of mental health; it is not the whole explanation, but it is a condition of possibility. The coercive and risk-averse character of statutory mental health services is seemingly an unpromising context for coproduction. However, the libertarian and anti-statist ideology of 'antipsychiatry' was a predictable reaction of dissent from those who entered medicine to help people rather than control them.

As for patients themselves, they too have not been of one voice. When the service user movement emerged in the 1970s in Europe and North America, it contained both reformist and abolitionist factions (Crossley, 2006). Now more dispersed and incoherent than in the past, that new social movement still contains those wanting to find new ways of working that are collaborative and those more suspicious or even dismissive of professional good intentions. Coproduction is favoured, then, by the reformist wing of the service users' movement, but others hold professional power in constant suspicion. Take the optimistic aspiration towards recovery (Anthony, 1993), which many user groups embrace and that is aligned with coproduction. Some user groups, such as Recovery in The Bin,[1] dismiss this policy trend angrily, reserving the right not to recover while demanding the obligation of state-employed professionals to respond to their expressed needs and that welfare benefits be aligned with the patient role. For some patients, though, the narrative of mental illness being a brain disorder associated with a chemical imbalance is accepted unreflectively. Many taking antidepressants see themselves as victims of this imbalance and are happy to embrace biomedical paternalism (e.g. Fullagar, 2009). This range of user perspectives suggest that a consensus about human agency is absent and their stance towards professional authority is highly mixed.

The above evidence of ambivalence in the policy, clinical and patient communities of interest affords a wide range of epistemological positions that might endorse coproduction optimistically or undermine it sceptically, or even cynically. We could stop at this point and limit our discussion of the prospects of coproduction to the linguistic matter of ideology, epistemology,

---

1. www.recoveryinthebin.org

discourse or competing perspectives. However, *ambivalence* at the collective or individual level within these communities of interest has emerged in part from external *ambiguities*. This matter of ontology, not just epistemology, can also be considered historically. What were the material as well as ideological conditions of possibility for coproduction to be both promoted but also constrained today?

One ontological frame of reference from critical realism that seeks to address that question is that of our four-dimensional social being. This refers to our relationship with nature, our relationship with one another, our relationship to our embedding socio-economic context and our individual and unique experience and character. Taking these one by one, I mentioned earlier that it may be the case that our cognitive impairments may be a function of bodily impairments. This has been the insistent position of the Kraepelinian biodeterminists. It is reductionist and largely unproven in terms of its neurological logic (mental disorders are deemed *ipso facto* to be brain disorders). The caution here, though, is that, notwithstanding that hoped-for reductionism, which has become part of the creed of mental health policy, we do not know for certain that it is wholly wrong in all cases. The arrogance of biodeterminism is no different from the arrogance of psychological or social determinism. In truth, when considering a complete grasp of why some people develop what are diagnosed as forms of mental disorder, we do not know for certain the answer, and so epistemic humility is implied.

Moreover, such a speculation is not required for some people already within the ambit of psychiatry (some of those with learning disabilities and all of those who are dementing), where there may be a clear organic basis to their psychological and social impairments. The prospects of coproduction with these groups necessarily requires a modified version of paternalism (advocates and supportive care workers). My point here is that our biology (part of the natural world) affords the *extent* to which we can act as human agents, mindful of what we want today and clear about future requirements. This does not negate the prospects of a version of coproduction, but it does require case-by-case consideration about its expected achievement and pragmatics.

Turning to the second ontological dimension, our relationality, coproduction implies sustained negotiations between professionals and clients. Indeed, coproduction is arguably *constituted* by relationality and so it may be tempting to ignore the other three dimensions listed. Coproduction is predicated upon the idea that good communication between mutually respectful parties will lead to an enhancement of service quality and a fuller recognition of the client's humanity and citizenship. This is an ideological assumption akin to that in industrial relations that all that is required is good communication and the ongoing opportunity to negotiate with our fellows. It is an assumption that may be warranted much of the time and is always open to testing out in practice. However, it *is* an assumption. It might be that there are irresolvable contradictions and constraints set by powers in the other three dimensions that undermine the prospects of success.

The third dimension (our embedding socio-economic norms) is about time and place. The emergence of coproduction was a function of the contradictions of the welfare state at the turn of this century, which I noted earlier. The welfare state both respects citizenship and selectively constrains it in the interests of social order and efficiency (Pilgrim, 2012). Moreover, it is difficult to turn the poor into *actual* consumers (the logic of the market) and psychiatric patients are overwhelmingly poor.

'Consumerism' has become necessarily distorted in healthcare more generally where service commissioners or purchasers now provide us with a newly emergent form of paternalism. They act on behalf of the local public and so heavily mediate a market relationship. This has required healthcare to become both marketised and more bureaucratised, with service performance being subjected to auditing. And *whose* needs are being responded to under conditions of marketisation and bureaucratisation? If psychiatric care is a 'service', then a service to whom? This ambiguity frames coproduction. For example, can the amalgam concept of 'users and carers' be the starting point for the non-professional dimension to coproduction? I would suggest that this is unwise, because the interests of users and their significant others may or may not be aligned.

The fourth dimension refers to our unique personalities. Some of us are happy to be dependent patients and would not be interested in the ethos of coproduction or any other prospect outside of that compliance with professional authority. Some of us fight for our personally preferred form of care (for example, acquiring a version of psychotherapy that suits us) but have little interest in the politics of the collective. Some of us have faith in service reform and the good will and good intentions of professionals, but some of us are nihilistic and distrust or scorn all professional authority. This range of personal positions is part of the context of the emergence and sustainability of coproduction.

Conclusion

In this short commentary, I have tried to place the content of the preceding chapters into a wider social and historical context. I have not commented on any chapter in particular, but the points I make above have resonances with them all in different ways. The ambivalence present between and within relevant communities of interest is an epistemological matter that can be addressed by forms of research on discourses and narratives. However, the ambiguity present in the material context of the latter also points to the need to address matters of biological, personal and social ontology. I introduced our four-dimensional social being frame of understanding from critical realism to enable that examination. Coproduction, like any topic to be researched, can be explored within and between those four planes of being.

References

Alford, J. (2009). *Engaging public sector clients: From service delivery to coproduction.* Palgrave.

Alford, R.R. (1975). *Health care politics: Ideological and interest group barriers to reform.* Chicago University Press.

American Psychiatric Association. (2013). *Diagnostic and statistical manual of mental disorders* (5th ed.). American Psychiatric Association.

Anthony, W.A. (1993). Recovery from mental illness: The guiding vision of the mental health system in the 1990s. *Psychosocial Rehabilitation Journal, 16*(4), 11–23.

Bean, P. (1980). *Compulsory admissions to mental hospitals.* Wiley.

Cohen, S. & Scull, A. (Eds.). (1983) *Social control and the state: Historical and comparative essays.* Basil Blackwell.

Crossley, N. (2006). *Contesting psychiatry: Social movements in mental health.* Routledge.

Double, D. (2007). Adolf Meyer's psychobiology and the challenge for biomedicine *Philosophy, Psychiatry & Psychology, 14*(4), 331–339.

Eastman, N. (1994). Mental health law: Civil liberties and the principle of reciprocity. *British Medical Journal, 308*(6920), 43–45.

Engel, G.L. (1980). The clinical application of the biopsychosocial model. *American Journal of Psychiatry, 137*(5), 535–544.

Fabris, E. (2011). *Tranquil prisons: Chemical incarceration under community treatment orders.* University of Toronto Press.

Fullagar, S. (2009). Negotiating the neurochemical self: antidepressant consumption in women's recovery from depression. *Health, 13*(4), 389–406.

Honneth, A. (1995). *The struggle for recognition: The moral grammar of social conflicts.* Polity Press.

Laing, R.D. (1966). *The politics of experience.* Penguin.

Macdonald, K. (1995). *The sociology of the professions.* Sage.

Martin, J.P. (1985). *Hospitals in trouble.* Blackwell.

Offe, C. (1993). *Structural contradictions of the welfare state.* MIT Press.

Pilgrim, D. (2012). The British welfare state and mental health problems: The continuing relevance of the work of Claus Offe. *Sociology of Health & Illness, 34*(7), 1070–1084.

Pilgrim, D. (2015). *Understanding mental health: A critical realist exploration.* Routledge.

Pilgrim, D. (2018). Are kindly and efficacious mental health services possible? *Journal of Mental Health, 27*(4), 295–297.

Riley, H., Fagerjord, G.L. & Høyer, G. (2018). Community treatment orders – what are the views of decision makers? *Journal of Mental Health, 27*(2), 97–102.

Sedgwick, P. (1982). *Psycho politics*. Pluto Press.

Szasz, T.S. (1963). *Law, liberty and psychiatry.* Macmillan.

Contributors

AB
After carefully exploring with AB the risks they might face if identified as co-author, we coproduced (with AB) the decision not to disclose any further information. We regret that they will forego the privileges associated with acknowledgement of publication that many of us may take for granted. We are, nonetheless, deeply grateful to AB for their contribution. We hope that one day it will be safe for all to express their views freely without fear of recrimination or unwanted media attention.

Don Bryant
Formerly a bank manager, with Midland Bank, Don Bryant set up a management training company with diverse clients across the north west of England. He then joined Imagine, a Liverpool-based mental health charity, before setting up an educational, training and employment centre for recovering drug users, which also made and installed 'alleygates' across the whole of Liverpool. Immediately before becoming ill with severe depression in 2008, he worked as operational manager for a domestic violence charity in Merseyside. Since 2009, he has acted in numerous capacities as a service user and carer representative, winning the Chairman's Award in 2015. He also served as a trustee of the national Mental Health Network (part of the NHS Confederation). He has always believed that if, as the NHS maintains, 'the patient is at the centre of everything we do', the patient must be involved in the decision-making processes, and he continues to fight that cause.

Mark Chandley
Mark Chandley has 38 years' experience as a mental health nurse. He has worked extensively on violence and aggression and has authored many texts on both this subject and on recovery and inclusion in mental health. He is a keen advocate

of socialism, fairness and equality. Both his degree and PhD were gained at the Manchester Metropolitan University under the tutorage of Emeritus Professor Joel Richman. He focused on an anthropological view of the world, largely ignoring psychiatry as a social construction and being more existential. With new eyes, he further posited some important socio-temporal questions about how both time and space is organised, focusing on Marx and Foucault as anchors by which to explore the world. He has toyed with antipsychiatry but believes there are flaws with this. Since then, he has lectured on various positive ways of managing extreme behaviours and again researched recovery in a high-secure setting, with all of its concomitant restraints and restrictive practices that should be simply eliminated in a modern health service. Currently, he is exploring the views of segregated patients with a view to developing new theory and writing about the digital revolution in industrial society. He is also working as a senior clinical nurse in Ashworth Hospital, encouraging debate and new theory.

Amanda Clayson

Amanda Clayson has a personal investment in 'recovery-based' research. She is exploring her own 'recovery journey' and working closely with others to explore theirs. She is the founder of VoiceBox Inc and is deeply committed to research driven by people with lived experience of the impacts of substance use. Amanda is a trained teacher, registered general nurse and a learning disability nurse. She has undertaken significant community development work integrating health, social care and learning. Her work brings together people with lived experience, research and practice, with the explicit aim of enhancing the reach and positive impact to people's lives. She has developed a rich 'toolbox' of approaches that harness the power of digital and creative media as vehicles for connection, capturing and communication of authentic voice. Her signature tool, 'VoiceBox', has been used in numerous academic and community contexts and has featured in academic journals and research conferences. She has extensive experience of participative action research in the areas of substance use, coproduction and inclusion, end-of-life care and community involvement in local authority decision-making. Amanda has published on participative methodology and critical reflections on coproduction. She has a commitment to dissemination beyond traditional academic approaches and has organised a number of community research festivals and street screenings of digital materials. She is a community research partner with Manchester Metropolitan University and an active member of the Substance Use and Associated Behaviour Research Group.

Rhiannon Corcoran

Rhiannon Corcoran is a professor of psychology and public mental health at the University of Liverpool. She has been researching mental health and wellbeing for 30 years and is particularly interested in how our spaces, places and communities impact us. She leads the community wellbeing evidence programme of the UK's What Works Centre for Wellbeing and co-directs the Prosocial Place Research and Practice Programme. From childhood, she has lived experience of caring for family members who have felt distressed. It is this experience, more than academic understandings, that has shaped how she approaches her work.

Albert Dzur

Albert W. Dzur is a democratic theorist interested in citizen participation and power-sharing innovations in education, criminal justice, healthcare and public administration. He is the author of *Democracy Inside: Participatory innovation in unlikely places* (2018); *Rebuilding Public Institutions Together: Professionals and citizens in a participatory democracy* (2017); *Punishment, Participatory Democracy, and the Jury* (2012), and *Democratic Professionalism: Citizen Participation and the Reconstruction of Professional Ethics, Identity, and Practice* (2008). He is a co-editor of *Democratic Theory and Mass Incarceration* (2016). His interviews with democratic innovators appear in *Boston Review*, *The Good Society*, the *International Journal of Restorative Justice* and *National Civic Review*. He is Distinguished Research Professor at Bowling Green State University.

Walid Elkharam

After completing his PhD on examining knowledge and adherence to health advice among adults with diabetes, at John Moores University, Walid Elkharam went back to his university in Libya and worked as an assistant professor of public health. As a result of the current situation in his country, he returned to the UK and, since 2017, has worked on a wide range of projects with NatCen Social Research, NHS and ARC/CLARHC NWC Research, which are focusing mainly on health promotion. He is passionate about being an advocate for people with long-term conditions and believes that coproduction is essential to improve healthcare services.

Anne Felton

As a mental health nurse, critical perspectives have underpinned Dr Anne Felton's practice as she maintained a commitment to finding different ways of working that challenge the power relationships within practice and the medicalisation of mental healthcare. Anne has carried these values into her academic role through the education of pre-registration mental health nurses and her research in the areas of decision-making, risk, coproduction and recovery. Anne is currently Head of Department at the Institute of Health and Allied Professions, Nottingham Trent University.

Pamela Fisher

Dr Pamela Fisher is an independent researcher. Until May 2019, she was a reader in social and health citizenship at Leeds Beckett University, having previously held academic posts at the universities of Sheffield, Huddersfield, Liverpool and Leeds. Her work offers critical sociological perspectives on resilience, wellbeing and mental health, particularly from the perspectives of marginalised and socially under-valued groups. She is interested in emerging forms of professionalism within health and social care that challenge traditional hierarchical relationships. Pamela led an Economic and Social Research Council-funded seminar series on mental health and coproduction, *Reimagining Professionalism in Mental Health: Towards coproduction*. The focus of the seminar series was authentic coproduction and how this might be realised through a fundamental re-imagining of the relationships between service users, carers and professionals.

Mike Hargreaves[1]

After carefully exploring with Mike Hargreaves the risks he might face if identified as co-author, we coproduced (with him) the decision not to disclose any further information. We regret that he will forego the privileges associated with acknowledgement of publication that many of us may take for granted. We are, nonetheless, deeply grateful to Mike for his contribution. We hope that one day it will be safe for all to express their views freely without fear of recrimination or unwanted media attention.

Elaine Harrison

Elaine Harrison is a single mother in her 50s, with a teenage daughter. She works from home as an internet trader. She has had a variety of jobs throughout her life, including secretary, home economist and financial adviser. She has experienced a deep depression and absolute euphoric moments in her life. She trained as a hypnotherapist/psychotherapist/counsellor in her late 30s. She is not a 'glass half empty person', and not even a 'glass half full'; her glass is full! She believes her life really did begin at 40. She enjoys writing, has a few projects on the go, and hopes to publish one day.

Stephen Joseph

Stephen Joseph trained as an adult and mental health nurse in Australia. He worked in mental health hospitals in Bendigo and Brisbane before moving back to London, where he worked in research teams into mental health and co-ordinated a charity supporting mental health service users in south west London. His PhD

---

1. The author's name has been changed to protect his identity.

in health and social care explored the tension between care and control in mental health services, focusing on the perception of control from the perspectives of African and Caribbean service users. He was also a lecturer in mental health law and leadership and management in healthcare in universities in the UK. He is currently working as a mental health clinician and researcher in Australia.

Frank Keating

Frank Keating trained as a social worker and his first position was in a large psychiatric hospital in Cape Town, South Africa. He continued to practise in mental health settings in South Africa and the UK. His doctoral studies explored the concept of cultural sensitivity in relation to mental health services in the UK. Frank evaluated a coproduction initiative to improve access to psychological therapies for Black and minority ethnic communities. He is currently Professor of Social Work and Mental Health in the Department of Social Work at Royal Holloway University of London.

Mick McKeown

Mick McKeown is Professor of Democratic Mental Health in the School of Nursing, University of Central Lancashire, and a trade union activist with UNISON, playing a role in union strategising on professional nursing. He has taken a lead in arguing the case for union organising to extend to alliance formation with service user/survivor groupings. He has published widely in the mental health field, including coediting the recent textbook, *Essentials of Mental Health Nursing*.

Catherine Mills

Catherine Mills has worked as service user and carer lead with Mersey Care NHS Foundation Trust since 2012. She is responsible for the engagement and involvement of service users and carers across Merseyside. Her interest in mental health originates in personal experience, as she has received services since 1996. Originally, she was involved with the trust as a service user. As her recovery journey progressed, she took up paid employment in 2012. Her work necessitates experience of coproduction in a variety of contexts. One such area is research, where she has been involved in several projects that have been coproduced with service users and carers. As a recipient of services and an employee, she is able to view issues from a dual perspective. She has engaged in coproduction as a service user and a staff member. She has always found coproduction rewarding, as it enables multiple skill sets to work together and gather in a range of perspectives. To her, it is a win-win scenario that nurtures positive relationships and prevents an 'us and them' situation from arising.

Andrew Passey

Andrew Passey's chapter relates to his PhD, which he undertook in the School of Health and Community Studies, Leeds Beckett University. His research examines the impacts of public service coproduction on professional staff, in contrast to much of the literature that instead tends to focus on the perspectives of service users and citizens. It involves critical policy discourse analysis, exploring the ways that economistic discourses have colonised the policy space and set limits to what local actors deem is possible when implementing policy. Micro-level research comprised semi-structured interviews, observation of meetings, analysis of locally produced texts, and thematic analysis. His work draws on theory from public management, economic sociology and the sociology of professionalism. Before his PhD, he worked as a policymaker in the civil service, including the Department of Health, as a researcher in the voluntary sector, and as a senior research fellow at the University of Technology in Sydney.

Shaun Peterson[2]

After carefully exploring with Shaun Peterson the risks he might face if identified as co-author, we coproduced (with him) the decision not to disclose any further information. We regret that he will forego the privileges associated with acknowledgement of publication that many of us may take for granted. We are, nonetheless, deeply grateful to Shaun for his contribution. We hope that one day it will be safe for all to express their views freely without fear of recrimination or unwanted media attention.

Kate Pieroudis

Kate Pieroudis joined the Social Care Institute for Excellence (SCIE) in 2018 and facilitates SCIE's Coproduction Network – the production of good practice materials about inclusion and coproduction and SCIE's coproduction training and consultancy. She curates and co-project manages National Coproduction Week. After graduating with a degree in neuroscience and psychology, she intended to become a clinical psychologist but discovered volunteering and community activism after volunteering on a youth exchange in Italy. She worked at the user-led organisation Action Disability Kensington & Chelsea for six years, in a range of policy and campaigning roles. She has 15 years' experience as a project manager and trainer, setting up the 'Back to Work' project at The Stroke Association, supporting stroke survivors into work or volunteering. Her project methodology and guides were incorporated into stroke services in Scotland and New Zealand. At Disability Rights UK,

---

2. The author's name has been changed to protect his identity.

she managed an award-winning national peer support project, 'Get Out Get Active', around disabled people and physical activity. She has a foundation in psychoanalytic psychotherapy from Arbours Association. As DJ Lil' Koko, she has a weekly show on Jazz FM called 'The Big Easy', showcasing the music and culture of New Orleans and shining a spotlight on marginalised music and voices.

David Pilgrim

David Pilgrim is Honorary Professor of Health and Social Policy at the University of Liverpool and Visiting Professor of Clinical Psychology at the University of Southampton. Now semi-retired, he trained and worked in the NHS as a clinical psychologist before completing a PhD in psychology and then a master's in sociology. With this mixed background, his career then split between clinical work, teaching and mental health policy research. His relevant publications include *Understanding Mental Health: A critical realist exploration* (2015); *Key Concepts in Mental Health* (5th ed.) (2019); *Child Sexual Abuse: Moral panic or state of denial?* (2018); and *Critical Realism for Psychologists* (2020).

Julian Raffay

Julian Raffay was working as Specialist Chaplain (Research, Education and Development) until his post at Mersey Care was cut in March and he was made redundant. Since then, he has completed his professional doctorate, exploring the relationship between mental health services and faith communities, with particular emphasis on the ethics of coproduction. He returned to church ministry as Interim Team Rector in the Four Saints team in Liverpool. He now works as Director of Chaplaincy Studies at St Padarn's Institute, where he leads a master's programme. Although he has avoided using mental health services, he has had his share of struggles over the years. He has found it an enormous privilege to be part of the editorial team of this book and to benefit from others' contributions. He has recently felt inspired by William Wilberforce and hopes that this book may contribute in its own way to the emancipation of service users, carers and staff from tyrannical bureaucracies.

Kris Southby

Kris Southby completed his PhD in May 2013, exploring the impact of football fandom on the social exclusion of adults with a learning disability. Following a career break in which he worked for the learning disability charity Mencap, Kris joined the Centre for Health Promotion Research at Leeds Beckett University as a research fellow. He has worked on various research projects and written broadly about health inequalities for socially disadvantaged groups. Kris's research generally uses participatory qualitative and creative methods to capture people's lived experience.

Gemma Stacey

Dr Gemma Stacey is a mental health nurse and associate professor at the University of Nottingham. Her research and practice are underpinned by a critical consideration of the organisational, relational and professional factors that influence the expression of values in healthcare practice. She is committed to the premise of healthcare education as a vehicle to promote emancipatory practice and has developed a programme of educational scholarship focused on approaches that enable transformational learning.

Maureen Thomas

Maureen (Mo) Thomas has lived all her life in the working class community of Bootle, Liverpool. Maureen is a strong believer in community solidarity and mutual support. She has used mental health services in the past and is committed to making changes that would improve the quality of care and provide better education and support for staff, which is so much needed. Maureen is concerned about climate change, recycling and reusing.

Michaela Thomson

Michaela Thomson has more than 25 years of experience of supporting people with learning disabilities in varying settings, the last 10 being in secure forensic services as a research practitioner. Before this, she was a social worker working in community services within deprived areas, again supporting people with learning disabilities and their families. She is committed to adopting a coproduced approach to her work, striving to meaningfully engage service users, carers and the public in a range of coproduced research-related activity involving the design, delivery and dissemination of research findings. Her focus throughout this remains firmly on the implementation of the most up-to-date evidence-based practice to best support the people who reside within the trust and their families and the staff teams who work alongside them. She believes the rising acknowledgement of coproduction and its benefits to those involved have facilitated this approach and contributed to a culture shift in the way services engage and interact with people. By sharing, developing and producing together, outcomes inevitably become more service user focused, which in turn develops pathways to recovery and rehabilitation. It was a privilege for her to coproduce their chapter with two service users from the trust. Both have a diagnosed learning disability, but they overcame all the challenges this posed to deliver this contribution and offer the reader ways in which coproduction can be developed and delivered, even in the most challenging of services.

Tim Thornton

Tim Thornton is Professor of Philosophy and Mental Health in the School of Nursing at the University of Central Lancashire. As well as contemporary philosophy of thought and language, his research mainly concerns conceptual issues in mental healthcare. He has published papers on clinical judgement, idiographic and narrative understanding, the interpretation of psychopathology and recovery. His books are *Wittgenstein on Language and Thought* (1998), *John McDowell* (2004, 2019), the co-authored *Oxford Textbook of Philosophy and Psychiatry* (2006) and the co-authored *Tacit Knowledge* (2013). He was a co-editor of the *Oxford Handbook of Philosophy and Psychiatry* (2014) and a senior editor of the journal *Philosophy, Psychiatry and Psychology*. He runs, with Gloria Ayob, a philosophy and mental health distance learning teaching programme at the University of Central Lancashire.

Michael Turner

Michael Turner is a disabled person who has been in the disability/service user field for most of his career. Most of his work has focused on involvement/coproduction and he has worked in a range of disabled people's organisations, other charities, universities and central and local government. He helped set up Shaping Our Lives, the national network of service users and disabled people, in the late 1990s and remains a member of its management committee. He worked in the coproduction team at the Social Care Institute for Excellence (SCIE) for eight years. He left SCIE in 2018 to combine part-time work at Merton Centre for Independent Living in south London with other work with other organisations, including Oxfordshire County Council and the Royal College of Occupational Therapists.

Lucy Webb

Lucy Webb is a mental health nurse and health psychologist, specialising in research into recovery in problematic substance use. Lucy has worked in child and adolescent psychiatry and drug and alcohol liaison as a senior nurse and team leader at St. George's Hospital, London. Trained in child and adolescent nursing, family therapy, creative therapies and groupwork, Lucy is a specialist practitioner in psychodynamic and cognitive interventions. This practice background has informed Lucy's interest in coproductive research that enables inclusion and meaningful service delivery, especially for communities and individuals who are reluctant to engage in mainstream healthcare. Lucy is an experienced researcher of service provision, engagement and service access for vulnerable adults and young people. She has conducted quantitative and qualitative research into care pathways and provision among substance users, and mental resilience among care leavers, and is currently working on international coproduction projects in Uganda and Brazil.

Julia Zielke

Julia Zielke is a lecturer in Sociology at CODE, a project-based start-up university in Berlin. She recently completed her PhD on relational approaches to wellbeing and wellbeing research at the University of Liverpool Management School, where she explored feminist and arts-based approaches to understanding wellbeing across multiple scales and in austere climates. Her academic writing is fuelled by her anger at not having had a language to talk about her own and her family's histories of depression, anxiety, borderline personality disorder and autism.

Name index

A

Abell, S. 120
Action Disability Kensington & Chelsea (ADKC) 128
Adkin, M. 175
Alford, J. 206
Alford, R.R. 208
Altschul, A. 192
American Psychiatric Association (APA) 209
Andrews, G.J. 79
Aneshensel, C.S. 166
Anteby, M. 164, 169, 171
Anthony, W.A. 210
Aristotle 149, 180
Arnstein, S. 3, 103
Asaba, E. 105
Atkinson, S. 78, 79

B

Bagnall, A.-M. 76–77
Bakhtin, M. 196
Banicki, K. 177, 179
Barker, P.J. 3, 178
Barnes, H. 185
Barnes, M. 197
Bartley, M. 66
Basaglia, F. 193
Baugh, W.H. 104
Bauman, Z. 190
Baxter, H. 4
Bean, P. 208
Beauchamp, T.L. 184
Becker, H. 52
Benefield, N. 195
Beresford, P. 131, 133, 167, 171

Berkes, F. 104, 112
Best, D. 105
Bion, W. 191
Blauvelt, A. 84, 85
Blom-Cooper, L. 46, 52
Boardman, J. 54
Bologh, R.W. 39
Bourdieu, P. 41
Bovaird, T. 163, 165, 167
Bowers, L. 91
Boyle, D. 105, 106, 112, 116
Brandsen, T. 164, 167–168
Brennan, D. 178
Bridges, T. 38
Brown, G.W. 78
Brownhill, S. 33
Bury, M. 37

C

Cabinet Office 32
Cahn, E. 43, 104, 135, 165
Calton, T. 196
Cameron, J. (Dir.) 13
Cameron, W.B. 179
Campbell, C. 78
Cappleman, R. 19
Care Programme Approach (CPA) 91–93, 95, 97
Care Quality Commission 32, 92
Carers Trust 98–99, 142
Carr, S. 28, 105, 133, 134, 135, 164, 165, 166, 167, 171, 172
Case, A. 198
Centre for Mental Health 50

Chambers, M. 9, 90, 91, 186
Chandley, M. 44, 45, 47
CHANGE 118
Chappell, A.L. 120
Chassot, C.S. 81
Childress, J.F. 184
Chockinov, H.M. 90
Church, K. 4, 194
Citizen's Advice 138
Clark, M. 28
Cleary, M. 90
Coffey, M. 44, 91–92, 199
Cohen, S. 52, 207
Comensus 150
Community Wellbeing Evidence Programme 76
Conder, J. 119
Cook, T. 117–118, 120
Cooke, A. 4
Cooper, D. 192
Coote, A. 105
Corcoran, R. 79, 86
Cornish, F. 78
Cottam, H. 86
Cox, N. 106
Cresswell, M. 192
Crick, T. 167
Critical Mental Health Nurses Network 193
Critical Psychiatry Network 193
Critical Values-Based Practice Network 19
Crossley, N. 193, 210
Crouch, C. 72

D

Davidson, N. 78
Davies, S. 32
Deaton, A. 198
Department of Health 4, 19, 32, 49, 91, 92, 94
Department of Health Learning Difficulties Research Team 120
Department of Health & Social Care 6, 46
Department of Health's National Research Strategy 120
Dickens, G. 97
Disabled People's Commission 133
Dodd, K. 61
Donaldson, L. 40
Double, D. 209
Douglass, F. 73

Duff, C. 79
Duncan, B.L. 178
Durkheim, E. 207
Durose, C. 105, 113, 165
Duxbury, J. 91
Dzur, A.W. 73, 90, 143, 191, 195, 197, 199

E

East London NHS Foundations Trust 157–158
Eastman, N. 209
Economic & Social Research Council (ESRC) 7, 106, 111, 112, 113
Edwards, A. 5
Emerson, E. 116
Engage 160–161
Engel, G.L. 209
European Monitoring Centre for Drugs and Drug Addiction (EMCDDA) 103
Evetts, J. 167, 171
Eyal, G. 167

F

Fabris, E. 208
Fallon, P. 46
Fernandez, A. 178
Ferrito, M. 44
Fiddler, M. 29
Fisher, M. 198
Fisher, P. 8, 40, 190, 196, 197, 200
Focht-New, G. 116
Foley, T. 185
Foot, J. 193
Ford, D. 16
Forman, M. (Dir.) 192
Forrest, S. 5, 14, 175, 178, 181, 182
Foucault, M. 48, 50, 184, 192
Francis, R. 5, 13, 176, 180–181
Frankena, T.K. 119
Freidson, E. 167
Fulford, K.W.M. 149, 150
Fullagar, S. 210

G

Gabriel, M. CBE 157
Garcia-Iriarte, E. 119
Gardiner, M.E. 194
Garfinkel, H. 46
George, S. 45
Gilbert, P. 14,

Gilbert, T. 120
Gilburt. H. 90
Glas, G. 72
Glynos, J. 105
Goffman, E. 44, 48, 192
Goodwin, N. 104
Gorman-Murray, A. 80
Gossop, M. 103
Grendon Underwood Prison 192
Griffiths, S.R. 183
Gurvitch, G. 45

H

Habermas, J. 73, 194
Haigh, R. 195
Hall, D.E. 180, 187
Halliburton, M. 67
Halligan, A. 40
Handy, C. 181–182
Hannigan, B. 91, 199
Hardy, R. 34
Harris, T. 78, 116
Harvey, D. 79
Hatton, C. 116
Hatzidimitriadou, E. 41
Health and Social Care Northern Ireland (HSCNI) 160, 161
Heller, J. 54
Herero, the 102
Hinings, C.R. 180
Hodgkinson, I.R. 168
Hodgkinson, S. 203
Honingh, M. 164, 167–168
Honneth, A. 37, 206
Horgan, A. 5
Horne, M. 105
Hubble, M. 5
Huckshorn, K.A. 91
Hui, A. 5
Hume, D 150
Hutchinson, A. 119
Hutchinson-Pascal, N. 131
Hutton Ferris, D. 195

I

Inglis, P. 117, 118, 120
Involvement Centre 19–24, 26–28
Ion, R. 72

J

James' Place 82
Jeffers, S. 58
Johnson, K. 120
Johnsson, L. 180, 182
Jones, M. 191

K

Kalathil, J. 40
Kara, H. 2, 16, 184
Kempster, S. 183, 184, 186
Kendall, T. 182
Kendell, R.E. 149
Kesey, K. 15, 52, 192
Keyes, C. 16
King's Fund 178
Kingsley Hall 192
Kitwood, T.M. 178
Kothari, A. 5–6
Kuh, D. 34

L

Laing, R.D. 192, 209
Laudet, A. 105
Leadbitter, J. 82
League of Friends 153
Lelliott, P. 90
Lencioni, P. 6
Levinas, E. 198
Lino, A.F. 167
Lived Experience Advisory Panel (LEAP) 14, 65
Liverpool John Moores University 159
Loeffler, E. 163, 165
Lovell, A. 119
Lukersmith, S. 176
Lwembe, S. 40

M

Macdonald, K. 207
MacIntyre, A. 149, 176, 178, 179–180, 182, 183, 184, 186
Mader, L.B. 170
Madlove: A Designer Asylum 82–83
Mad Pride 192
Mad Studies 192
Main, T. 191
Marmot, M.G. 78
Martin, J.P. 207

Marx, K. 52
Mason, T. 45, 47, 49, 96
Massey, D. 80
Mauws, M.K. 180
May, N. 5–6
May, R. 184
McCallum, A. 3–4, 5, 9
McDonald, K.E. 118, 119
McKeown, M. 45, 51, 71, 95, 97, 98, 194
Mencap 120
Mendes, F. 81
Mental Health Consortium 159
Mental Health Foundation 170
Mental Health Network 154, 155
Mental Health Taskforce 166
Mental Patients Union (MPU) 192
Mercer, D. 45
Mersey Care NHS Foundation Trust (MCNHSFT) 85, 89, 92–95, 97, 99
Mersey Care's Spirituality Lived Experience Advisory Panel 14
Meyer, A. 209
Mid Staffordshire NHS Trust 5, 13, 176, 180–181
Mill, J.S. 207
Millett, K. 192
Mind 202
Monderman, H. 81
Moore, G. 67, 176, 180, 181, 182, 186
Moore, M.H. 166
Mo's House 81–82
Mudhoni, C. 3–4

N

N8/ESRC 106, 111, 112, 113
Nash, C.J. 80
National Development Team for inclusion (NDTi) 135, 202–203
National Institute of Health Research (NIHR) 81, 159, 160
National Institute of Health Research's School for Social Care Research (NIHR-SSCR) 32
Nedopil, N. 45
Needham, C. 28, 105
Newbigging, K. 93
New Economics Foundation (NEF) 3, 84, 90, 202
NHS Confederation 154

NHS England 97
NHS Foundation Trust 157–158
NHS Race and Health Observatory 158
NHS R&D North West 159
Norfolk and Suffolk NHS Foundation Trust 158
Northway, R. 120

O

Offe, C. 207
Oliver, K. 5–6
Olson, M.E. 196
Open Dialogue 196
Oppenheimer, J.R. 54
Orwell, G. 47
Os, J.V. 5
Osborne, S.P. 164, 168, 169, 170
Ostrom, E. 73, 84, 104, 163
Ostrom, V. 73

P

Palumbo, R. 28
Parsons, T. 49
Pascoe, C.J. 38
Patel, M. 134
Pennington, A. 77
Penny, J. 90
Peplau, H. 175, 176, 181
Perkins, R. 143
Philadelphia Association 192
Pickett, K. 78
Pieroudis, K. 127, 138, 139
Pilgrim, D. 44, 48, 72, 165, 166, 168, 208, 210, 212
Pine II, B.J. 5
Podogrodzka, M. 185
Prilleltensky, I. 79
Prilleltensky, O. 79
Proctor, H. 192
Proctor, N. 96
Psichiatria Democratica (Democratic Psychiatry) 193
Public Health England 103

Q

Quadara, A. 96
Quirk, A. 90

R

Raffay, J. 7, 15, 67, 175, 177, 178, 180, 181, 183, 186
Rawls, J. 194
Reader Organisation, The 83
Recovery in The Bin 192, 210
Recovery in Action 74,
Recovery Voice in Action 74, 104, 106, 111, 113
Reid, L. 79
Repper, J. 143
Research Excellence Framework (REF) 112
Reville, D. 4
ReVision 159
Richardson, L. 165
Richman, J. 458
Riley, F. 43
Riley, H. 208
Robert, G. 28
Roberts, G. 54
Roberts, M. 72
Robinson, M. 34
Rogers, A. 72
Rosanvallon, P. 194
Rose, D. 40, 143
Rose, N. 78
Rotheram, C. 186
Royal College of Psychiatrists 185
Royal Voluntary Service 153
Russo, J. 193

S

Salisbury Centre for Mental Health 31
Salpêtrière (asylum) 54
Salvador-Carulla, L. 176, 182
San, the 102, 103, 104
Santayana, G. 147
Sartre, J.-P. 45
Schalock, R.L. 115–116
Schizophrenia Commission 5, 13, 67, 175, 180, 182, 183, 186
Schön, D.A. 4
School of Analytical and Cognitive Hypnotherapy (SACH) 60
Scottish Recovery Network 43
Scull, A. 207
Schumacher, E.F. 67
Sedgwick, P. 2, 148, 192–193, 194, 198, 199–200, 207

Seedhouse, D. 184
Seikkula, J. 196
Sellman, D. 180, 183
Sequeira, H. 116
Sheffield's Spirituality Strategy Group 7
Shepherd, A. 53
Shils, E. 44, 45–46
Shine, B. 60
Shippee, N. 105
Silva, E. 53
Skellern, E. 192
Slay, J. 3, 5, 13, 31, 90, 165, 166, 175, 176, 202
Smith, T.S. 79
Social Care Institute for Excellence (SCIE) 74, 127–130, 137–139
Social Research Association 111
Social Work Action Network 193
Soteria Network 83
Spandler, H. 192, 193, 194
Speed, E. 105
Spirituality Lived Experience Advisory Panel (Mersey Care) 14
Springham, N. 28
Stacey, G. 19, 196
Stack, E. 119
Staniszewska, S. 4, 19, 67
Steen, T. 171–172
Stephens, L. 3, 5, 13, 31, 165, 166, 175, 176, 202
Stickley, T. 5
Storm, M. 5
Suarez-Balcazar, Y. 105
Sullivan, M. 38, 176, 178, 184, 185, 187
Sullivan, W. 186, 187
Survivors History Group 7
Survivors Speak Out 192
Swan, T. 52
Sweeney, A. 130, 190, 193
Swinton, J. 183, 185
Szasz, T 149, 192, 209

T

Taggart, D. 198
Taleb, N. 180
Taylor, P. 52
The Vacuum Cleaner 82, 83
The Reader Organisation 83
The Retreat 54, 191
Thiel, J.J. 80

Thomas, M. 81–82
Thrift, N. 80
Tilt, R. 46
Toth, G. 81
Townsend, P. 78
Tritter, J. 3, 4, 5, 9
Tuurnas, S. 164, 167, 171–172
Tyszkowska, M. 185

U

UK Drug Policy Commission 103
UN Committee Against Torture (UNCAT) 49, 54
UN General Assembly 49
University of Liverpool 159

V

VoiceBox 74, 106–107, 109, 216
Voices from the Brink 107
Völlm, B. 45

W

Wall, L. 95
Walmsley, J. 120
Walsh, J. 7, 176
We Coproduce 134
Wehrens, R. 106
What Works Centre for Wellbeing 76–77
Whicher, A. 167
White, S.C. 79
White, W.L. 105
Wilkinson, R. 78
Williams, B.N. 169, 172
Winship, G. 192
Wolfensberger, W.P. 116
Wonders, S. 177
World Health Organization (WHO) 113
WRVS 153
Wulf, W. 80

Y

Young, I.M. 194

Z

Zielke, J. 82

Subject index

A

abuse
  of people with learning disabilities 116
  in psychiatric system 72, 192, 207
  racist, 34
access (*see also* involvement)
  to care plans 97
  to mental healthcare 36, 41, 143
    for people with learning disabilities 120
  national targets for, 181
accessible information 118, 119, 142
advance directives 91
agency 8, 14, 40, 67
  constraints on, 166, 167
  loss of, 199
  patient, 178–179, 183, 191, 196
  role in recovery 89
    for black men 33, 34, 38–39
  of staff 179, 184
antipsychiatry 178, 182, 192–193, 207, 209–210
Art of Coproduction: A guerrilla guide, The (We Coproduce) 134
Asylum: The magazine for democratic psychiatry 193
Asylum: The radical mental health magazine 193
austerity 4, 49, 186, 193
  politics of, 72, 78

B

barriers (*see also* communication, access, values)
  to coproduction 130–138
    framework for understanding, 143
    solutions to, 138–140
  lack of funding as, 108
  systemic, in mental health services 27, 40, 197
biodeterminist/ism 209, 211
bioethics 183, 184
biomedical
  definitions of mental distress, 4
  ethics 178
  model 167, 185
  paternalism 210
  psychiatry 143
  treatments 45, 209
biopsychological model 178, 209
black men
  mental health of, 31–32
  in the mental health system 31ff
  and recovery 32–34
    collaboration and, 40–41
    model for, 34–39
Black Report, The 78
bottom-up change 26, 29
  coproduction as, 105, 158
  influences 111

C

capacity
  -building 161
  human, for pro-social relations 81
  mental,
    of people with learning disabilities 119, 121
    reflexive, of professionals 172
  of services/professionals, to support

coproduction 136, 172
    of service users 5, 19, 93, 94, 142
capability-building approach 86
care planning (*see also* Triangle of Care)
    carers' role 142
    and coproduction 89ff
    in dementia care 93–94
    in forensic settings 95–98
    in inpatient mental healthcare, 93
    recovery-oriented principles in, 96–97
carer(s)
    distinct needs of, 212
    involvement of,
        in care process 98, 130, 142
        in service design and planning 157, 186
    potential role in coproduction 5, 74, 132–133, 184, 202
    power imbalance 20
    professionals' attitudes to, 14–15
    support for, in caring role 97–98
    training for, 158
    valuing, by trusts 153
    views of the mental health system 19–20
carer and service user assembly 154
chaplains 175
citizen-consumer 105
citizen engagement 165
collaboration 40
    challenges of, in secure care 45, 47, 52, 96
    peer (men's groups) 40–41
co-creation 172
    events 32, 33
    value, 168–170, 171
coercion (*see also* involuntary treatment)
    arguments in defence of, 209
    incompatibility with coproduction 168
    legitimisation of, 47, 190
coercive
    interventions/practice 34, 45, 48, 49, 80, 91
    mental health law 208
    power of state 165
    social control 52, 207
    system of mental healthcare 193, 210
commissioners
    'paternalistic', 212
    role in coproduction 112, 202
communication
    barriers to,
        with carers 21
    overcoming, with people with learning disabilities 121
    competition vs, 203
    deliberative democratic, 196
    enhancement by coproduction 166
    facilitation of, with service users 94
    importance of, in coproduction 133, 140
    power of turbulent, 194
    and relationality 211
    and social democratic processes 194, 195, 203
    within families 98
compliance
    collective, 52–53
    with 'dominant truths' 47
    with protocols 40
    with treatment 33, 98, 212
Connecting and Realising Value through People (Engage) 160
consensus
    in coproduction 23, 29, 85, 186
constraints
    on coproduction 143, 166–167, 172, 196
    on democratic professional practice 197
    on user/carer involvement 26
consultation
    in coproduction 104, 112
    as distinct from coproduction 129, 131
    in research, with people with learning disabilities 123
consumer
    feedback 182, 206
    mental patient as, 212
consumerism
    in healthcare 5, 212
    in the welfare state 208
contextual knowledge 182
co-operation 16, 43
    in approach to care 91–92, 95, 96, 98
    and co-option 194–195
    as human tendency 79
    with 'out groups' 85
co-option 206
    challenging, 163ff
    of coproduction 148
coproduction
    ethical imperative for, 130
    fear of, 135–136
    involuntary, 169

legal requirement for, 130
in research 111–112
benefits of, 121
social benefits of, 105
tokenistic, 78, 131, 153
voluntary, 170–171
critical realism 211

D

decision-making
levelled up, 83
shared, 20, 22, 72, 196
in coproduction 28, 104, 160, 161
forums for, 18–19
impacts of, 77
in secure settings 98
strategies for, 128
deliberative democracy 80, 194, 195, 196
Dementia Reconsidered: The person comes first (Kitwood) 178
democracy 72, 148, 194–196
in coproduction 190, 196–197
impediments to, 203–204
deficiencies of, 190
illusion of, 156
in relationships of care 193
democratic
political activism 194
practices 190, 196
professionals 71, 73, 197
democratisation
calls for, from survivor/users 73
of mental healthcare 3, 71, 200
of space 73, 84
staff commitment to, 157
democratised
care 143, 191, 196
psychiatry 199
services 143
settings 192
social relations 148, 191
space 81
descriptive claims (*see also* normative claims) 150
design
biophilic, 86
co-, 86, 161, 170, 183
coproduction as, 90, 127, 164, 165, 167, 170, 202, 203

democratised, 73
prosocial, 142
detainment 48, 49, 50, 51, 54, 133, 166
Diagnostic and Statistical Manual of Mental Disorders (APA) 209
dissent 52, 195, 210
doctor(s) 26, 51, 78, 175
Dragons' Den 62

E

EastEnders 64
Easy Read leaflets 74, 117, 118, 121, 123, 138, 142
'embedding' 134, 161, 202, 211, 212
Embedding Co-production in Mental Health 202
employability 166
empowerment 79, 96, 196, 206
as outcome of coproduction 43, 121, 124, 163
enabler(s)
coproduction as, 160
for coproduction 143
engagement
community, in recovery 105
in coproduction 28, 134, 169
factors that promote/prevent, 40, 90
family, in care planning 97
public/civic, 23, 128, 195
with others/groups 38
in research 120–121, 122, 123, 124
with treatment/services 103, 165
user, legitimising effect 167
Enlightenment, the 184
ethical review (research) 131
ethics
biomedical, 178
of coproduction 6, 184–185
principles of, 184–185, 186
organisational, 180
of rationality 198
of responsibility 198
virtue, 180, 184, 186, 187
ethical
arguments for coproduction 175, 178, 179–180
challenges
in forensic settings 66–67
in research with people with learning

disabilities 119
imperative for coproduction 130
oversight (in research) 110, 111
procedures (in research) 106, 110
review (in research) 131

F

facilitated space
  importance to coproduction 172
facilitation
  and co-option 172
  of research tasks 172
  of social engagement 37
facilitators
  policy and legislation as, 142
  professionals/staff as, 133
faith communities 15, 177, 179, 184, 185, 186
Francis Report, The 180

H

harm
  due to mental health system 5, 47, 194, 196
  due to work 50
  risk of, from coproduction 66
  self-, 5
harmony
  of relational approach 86
  social and physical, 87
  in wellbeing 180, 187
Health Gap, The (Marmot) 78
Heart and Soul of Change, The (Duncan et al.) 178
How to Make Information Accessible (CHANGE) 118
human trafficking 148, 175

I

Ideal Ward Round project 19ff
implementation
  authenticity of, in coproduction 199
  of Ideal Ward Round project 21, 23, 28
  'key steps to coproduction' 161
individualism
  vs collaboration 39–41
  cult of, 72
  vs relational 38, 39
inequalities
  health and social, 16
  in mental health 40
  race, 31–32
  socio-economic, 78, 86
involuntary (*see also* coercion, voluntary)
  coproduction 169
  involvement of public service users 164–165
  treatment 48, 208
interpretative phenomenological analysis 33
involvement
  payment for, 128, 138, 153
  of people with learning disabilities 137–138
  public, 103, 163, 164
    and research 159–160
  in service development forums 118, 129
  tokenistic, 77

J

'Just and Learning Culture' policy 157

K

Kalahari desert 102, 104
Kraepelinian tradition 209, 210, 211

L

learning disability/ies
  forensic settings 115ff
LGBTQI 130
life-story work 94
lived experience
  researchers with, 108
  shared, importance of 35
  staff with, 7
  value of, to coproduction 140, 160, 161, 166, 184
Loony Bin Trip, The (Millett) 192

M

Mandela rules 49, 54
Marxians 207
medicalisation
  of mental health problems 133
men's groups (black) 40–41
mental distress 191, 195
  links with capitalism 198
  as sign of weakness 37
Mental Health Act 1983 26, 32, 50, 54, 90, 93, 208

Code of Practice 46, 94
Mind Magic (Shine) 60
Mind Waves (Shine) 60

N

neoliberal/ism 72, 78, 79, 83, 167, 171, 195, 196, 198, 199
New Public Management 166, 171, 196
NHS constitution 6, 52
Nineteen Eighty-Four (Orwell) 47
No More Throw-Away People (Cahn) 135
normative claims 150
nurses 13, 14, 19, 47, 93, 160, 175, 180, 181

O

obstacles to change 72–73
occupational therapists 175
One Flew Over the Cuckoo's Nest (Kesey) 192

P

participatory approaches 71, 199
paternalism
  medical, 4, 67, 207
  state, 207, 209–211, 212
peer support/networks 96, 105, 123, 129, 133, 160
  black, 31, 33, 34, 37, 40
  educators (children) 170
  researchers 130
  services 161
Peppa Pig 65
performance measures 166
person-centred care 20, 142, 148–149, 209
political
  activism 194
  alliances 3, 73
  context 78, 82, 148, 198, 209
  coproduction as, 4
  mental health as, 192–193, 194, 198
positive-sum power 165
power-sharing 132–134
Poynton Regenerated [video] 81
Principles of Biomedical Ethics (Beauchamp & Childress) 184
processes
  care, 20, 91–92
    as alienating, 193
  coproduction, 77, 168–170, 172, 191
  decision-making, 77, 128
  democratic, 91, 171, 194
  ethical (research), 130–131
  public, 83
  relational design, 84
  reparative, of psychiatric harms 194
  research, 106, 108, 110, 111, 112, 119, 120, 159
  risk-management, 46, 47
  social, 5
procedures
  care, 153
  coproduction, 155, 202
  ethical, 106, 110
professionalism 40, 90,
  democratic, 193
  as exclusivity 143
  relationality and, 164, 167, 171, 172
psychiatry
  biomedical/biological, 143, 148, 209, 211
  democratic tendencies in, 191–194
  fear of, 34, 209
  legitimacy of, 72–73
  relational challenge to, 195, 196
  secure, 49
  transforming, 198–199
Psycho Politics (Sedgwick) 192
psychosocial interventions 98,
public
  inquiry/ies 46, 176
  management 164
  mental health 78
  safety 72, 81, 99
  service 72
  services 72, 73
    coproduction in, 84, 106, 112, 136, 143, 148, 163, 164–165, 167, 168, 170–171
  spaces 80
  value, coproduction as contributor to 168–170, 171

Q

quality assurance committee 154, 155

R

R factor framework 107–111
recovery 5, 72
  alternatives to model 185
  of black men 31ff
    culture, role of 40

and identity 40
  model of, 34–39, 41
  outside statutory services 39–40
  study of coproduction and, 32–34
care planning and, 91–92, 95–96
co-option of, 131–132
critics of model 210
language, as barrier to coproduction 110
personal agency and, 89–90
as an R factor 108–109
relational spaces and, 80–83, 195–196
risk and, 46–47, 48, 54
as social movement 105
as threshold for withdrawal of services 167
Recovery Star 97
Recovery Voice in Action project 74, 106–107, 111, 113
Recovery Walk (Manchester) 104
regulation
  clinical governance 40
  statutory, 180, 182
relational (*see also* recovery, professionalism, psychiatry)
  aspects of care planning 92
  boundaries 177
  care 143, 148, 191–192
  competence/skills 171–172, 196
  design 83–86
  nature of coproduction 14, 211, 169
  nursing practices 28
  security 49
  services 193–194
  spaces 80–86, 142
  tools for change 193–194, 199
  wellbeing 73, 78–79, 81–8
    arts and, 82–83
relationality, in public services 194–195, 198
relationships
  in care planning 98
  central to coproduction 9, 14–15, 28, 40, 59, 107, 132, 133–134, 135, 161, 169
  democratisation of, 3, 71, 72, 191, 193, 194, 196
  doctor–patient, 26
  re-traumatising, 198
  role in recovery 33, 34, 36–37, 38, 39, 40–41
  in secure settings 95

intimate, 51–48, 50
mutual, 43–44, 45, 48, 49, 51–52
power and, 52–53
with service providers 40
trusting, 31, 85
and wellbeing 77–78
research
  action learning, 129
  coproduced, 105–106,
    lack of, 119–120
    tips for, 121–122
  emancipatory, 119
  facilitated collaborative action, 117
  participatory, 105, 119–120
  strategy, national 120
resilience
  as benefit of coproduction
    to individuals 166
    to mental health services 170
  black men's 37
resistance
  to coproduction 72, 98, 135, 156, 203
  to the mental health system 195, 200
restraint
  control and, 32, 96
restrictive
  environments 190,
  practices 46, 48–49, 52, 53, 90, 91, 135, 216
reusable learning object (RLO) 24
right 'not to recover' 210
Rise of Coproduction, The [Blog] 203
risk
  at-risk patient/service user/groups 92, 119, 199
  -averse/aware system 72, 74, 132, 140, 203, 210
  management 40, 44, 50, 199
    in secure services 90, 91, 92, 94, 95, 99
  presented by coproduction 109, 134, 135, 140, 163
  and recovery 46–47
  -taking 85, 109, 111

S

safe spaces
  for black men 34–36, 39
seclusion 47, 49, 54, 96
segregation 44, 48, 49, 54, 55, 133, 191

social
  context 32, 169, 191, 207
  inclusion 8, 33, 185
  workers 128, 160, 175
socio-economic
  context 211
  inequalities 78, 86
  norms 212
socio-politics 79
spirituality 176, 177, 178, 183, 186
stigma
  and drug use 103
  mental health, 44, 49, 53, 83, 108, 166, 185–186, 199
    and black men 33, 36, 37, 41
  reduction in, 86, 109
substance use(rs) 33, 108
  access to services 103–104
survivor
  activism 191
  groups 49, 194
  movement(s) 7, 71, 73, 81, 87, 194, 197
  voices 197

T

The Dark Side of Coproduction (Kothari & May) 4
therapeutic
  alliance(s) 90, 96
  communities 191–192, 195
  outcomes 16
  relationships 3, 6, 22, 33, 194, 198
    lip service to, 49
time banking 104, 136
Titanic (film) 13, 14
trade unions 73, 197
  alliance with survivor groups 194
trauma
  effects of, 190, 198
  -informed care 54, 95–96, 198
  racialised, 37, 41
  social, 195
Triangle of Care 74, 98
Triangle of Care 98, 99, 142

V

values
  African, 38
  collective, 105
  coproductive, 29, 104, 116, 127, 129, 132, 133, 134, 140, 150, 161, 165, 184
  in mental health 179–183
  in mental healthcare 149–150
  of NHS constitution 52
  prejudiced, 102
  shared, 34
  Western, 177
virtue ethics 180, 184, 186, 187
vision
  shared, in coproduction 130
VoiceBox 106–107
voluntarism 208

W

ward round(s) 18, 19, 26
  Ideal Ward Round project 18ff
  recommendations for improving, 20–21, 29
wellbeing
  co-creating, 185–186, 199
  community, 38
    involvement 76–78
  of patients/users 40
  physical spaces and, 80, 82, 83
  recovery and, 105
  relational, 73, 78–79, 83–87
  scale 16
  social/emotional, 39, 168
    of children 170

X

X Factor, The 62

Z

'Zero Suicide' policy 157
zero sum 143, 148, 165